LIZ EARLE'S
QUICK GUIDES
Acne

LIZ EARLE'S
QUICK GUIDES

Acne

B☘XTREE

Advice to the Reader
*Before following any advice contained in this book, it is
recommended that you consult your doctor if you suffer from any health
problems or special condition or are in any doubt.*

First published in Great Britain in 1995 by Boxtree Limited,
Broadwall House, 21 Broadwall, London SE1 9PL

Copyright © Liz Earle 1995
All rights reserved

The right of Liz Earle to be identified as Author of this Work has
been asserted by her in accordance with the Copyright, Designs and
Patents Act 1988

10 9 8 7 6 5 4 3 2 1

ISBN: 0 7522 1631 7

Text design by Blackjacks
Cover design by Hammond Hammond

Except in the United States of America this book is sold subject to the
condition that it shall not, by way of trade or otherwise, be lent,
resold, hired out or otherwise circulated without the publisher's prior
consent in any form of binding or cover than that in which it is
published and without a similar condition including this condition
being imposed upon a subsequent purchaser

Printed and Bound in Great Britain by Cox & Wyman Ltd,
Reading, Berkshire

A CIP catalogue entry for this book is available from
the British Library

Contents

Acknowledgements 6

Introduction 7

1 What is Acne? 9

2 Conventional Treatments for Acne 25

3 A Natural Approach 39

4 The Anti-Acne Diet 53

5 Clear Skin Care 69

Glossary 83

Useful Addresses 87

Index 89

Acknowledgements

I am grateful to Michelle Pamment for helping to produce this book. Also my thanks to Dr Nicholas Lowe of 15 Harley Street, London and Clinical Professor of Dermatology at UCLA, Santa Monica, USA; dermatologist and founder of the Acne Support Group Dr Anthony Chu, and researcher Sarah Hamilton-Fleming. I am also indebted to the talented team at Boxtree, and to Rosemary Sandberg and Claire Bowles Publicity for their unfailing enthusiasm and support.

Introduction

Acne affects 40 percent of the population at some point in their lives. This frightening statistic is virtually more than for any other disease known to man. Yet acne is still not taken seriously as a medical disability by some. Unfortunately, acne first strikes during puberty – a time of raging hormones and unsettled emotions. It can be a significant cause of lost confidence, social problems and teenage angst. Unlike other ailments, acne is hard to hide. Facial spots and pimples can be a real disability when it comes to achieving success with first dates or even college and career interviews.

Fortunately, acne is a treatable condition. There is no reason why any young person should grow up traumatised by poor skin or scarred by acne pitting. The key is to catch the symptoms early on. A visit to a sympathetic (and informed) GP, possibly followed by a referral to a dermatologist or skin specialist, is essential. Many different treatments exist to treat acne for both boys and girls, in the young and even the middle-aged. If acne is affecting your life, or the life of a relative or friend, please read this *Quick Guide*. Learn what can be done to control the condition and seek expert medical attention before the skin is scarred for life. Even if your skin is bad and you believe there is no hope, there is a great deal that can be done to minimise the damage and give your complexion the best chance of looking good.

Liz Earle

1

What is Acne?

Acne vulgaris, the medical name for acne, appears on approximately 80 percent of teenagers at some point in time, as well as on a large number of adults. It is an inflammatory disorder of the skin, consisting of blackheads, spots, greasy skin and, in severe cases, scarring and cyst-like eruptions. While far from being a life-threatening condition it can, for some people, feel like a life-wrecking one, and the resulting scars are not just confined to the physical. Dr Anthony Chu, leading dermatologist and founder of the Acne Support Group, says that even some of his patients are not totally aware of the effect that their acne has on them and a common remark following successful treatment is: 'I never fully realised the person I could be until the acne was eventually cleared from my skin.'

Any problems we have with our skin may seem all the more harrowing because it's the first thing that people see. How many times have you heard people say they can't leave the house because they've got a huge spot on their nose or a rash on their face? And in a society that places such importance on physical beauty, a skin condition like acne can be emotionally destructive. Studies conducted in the USA have shown that people with acne scored badly in tests for anxiety, depression and well-being, even when compared to those suffering from debilitating diseases.

There is some good news, though. There are steps you can take to control your acne which range from using over-the-counter creams and prescription antibiotics to following a thorough cleansing routine, making dietary changes and using appropriate cosmetics and concealers.

How the Skin Functions

Acne is the most common of all skin problems but, before examining the causes of this skin condition, it is important to understand the function of our skin and how it's constructed. The skin is the body's largest organ, measuring two square metres in area and weighing between four and six pounds. It is a tough, self-repairing, flexible cover for the body that holds all our other bits together and it is the body's first line of defence, making sure that foreign bodies stay on the outside and essential fluids on the inside. After the brain, it is the body's most active and complicated organ, made up of literally thousands of different components, including sweat glands, oil-producing (sebaceous) glands, blood vessels, nerve endings, sensory cells, heat and cold receptors, touch receptors, hairs and muscles. The skin regulates temperature, excretes waste products through sweat, passes on feelings of pleasure through touch and warns of potential pain. Our skin even helps us attract members of the opposite sex by excreting a musk-like odour.

The skin displays varying characteristics in different areas of the body, depending on the particular requirements of those areas. For example, the cheeks have a soft, smooth surface while the forehead and nose are oilier. The skin on the palms, soles and fingertips have specialist surfaces which produce very little grease but a greater amount of moisture.

The skin is also an effective barometer of our health and well-being – a mirror of the internal condition of the body, providing indicators of what's happening within. In some Eastern cultures there is a system of diagnosing illnesses which is based solely on the texture, colour and odour of the skin. If you are feeling fit and healthy and on top of the world, the chances are that your skin will glow. But if you're ill or just generally run down, your skin may be dull in pallor or you may break out in spots. Severe nutritional deficiencies will be

WHAT IS ACNE?

reflected pretty quickly in our skin, as low levels of nutrients will be redirected to other parts of the body, such as the vital organs, where they are needed more urgently.

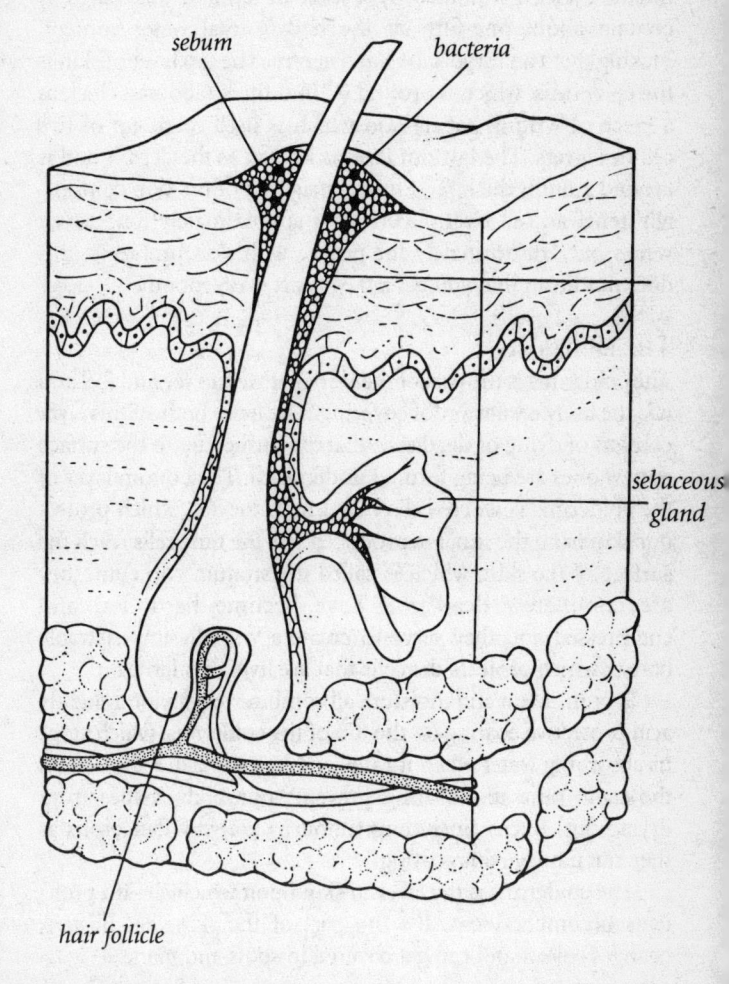

sebum

bacteria

sebaceous gland

hair follicle

Structure of the Skin

There are two main layers of skin, which rest on top of our muscle system, separated by a layer of fat, and together they contain about one-fifth of the body's total water content, making them an important water centre. The top layer of skin is the epidermis, which is around 0.2mm thick (about as thick as a piece of writing paper) and which is itself made up of five cellular layers. The bottom layer is known as the dermis and is around 1.8mm thick. The upper structure of the skin continually renews itself over a period of approximately four to six weeks but, unfortunately for people with skin problems, this does not mean that you get a fresh start every month.

THE EPIDERMIS

The epidermis is the part of the skin that we can see and feel and it is the body's waterproof covering. The main body of this layer consists of dying or dead cells that are pushed up to the surface as new ones are being formed underneath. The bottom layer of the epidermis is where cells called melanocytes, which protect our skin from the sun, are produced. By the time cells reach the surface of the skin, which is called the stratum corneum, they are completely dead and have become hard, flat and compressed and they serve to create a virtually impenetrable barrier which protects the cells that are living underneath.

Sebum, sweat and moisture all combine to provide a slightly acid protective coating on the top of the epidermis, which stops us absorbing water when it rains or when we take a shower. At the same time this coating prevents our body tissues from drying out. Burns (including sunburn) are very dangerous as they can damage this coating.

The epidermis is the layer of skin upon which all skin problems become evident. It's the part of the skin that blisters, changes colour and can get covered in spots and marks.

WHAT IS ACNE?

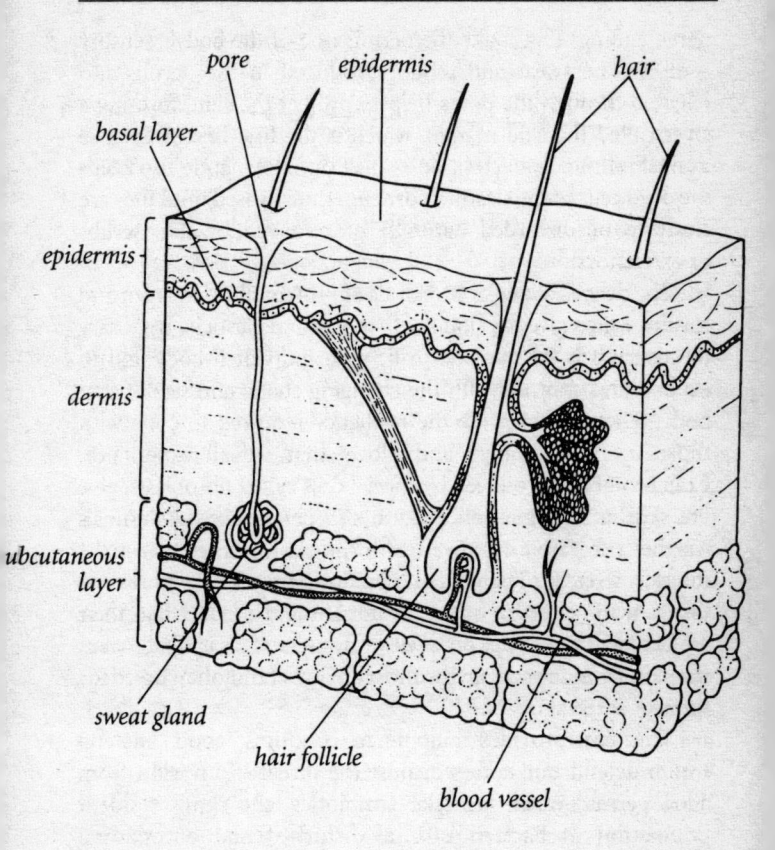

pore, epidermis, hair, basal layer, epidermis, dermis, subcutaneous layer, sweat gland, hair follicle, blood vessel

THE DERMIS

Lying beneath the epidermis is a thicker layer – the dermis. Its function is to support and feed its partner, the epidermis, via blood capillaries and the lymphatic system that is essential to feed and remove waste from the new skin cells. It also contains important features of its own such as sebaceous glands (these are bigger on the facial, shoulder and neck areas of the body), sweat glands that control our temperature, hair follicles and the nerve endings that make the dermis one of the body's sensory centres. The sweat and sebum produced in the dermis and released through the pores help to protect the skin, forming a layer called the acid mantle, which is the first line of defence against unfriendly bacteria and infection. The mantle also keeps the dead cells in the stratum corneum moisturised until they are ready to be discarded naturally or removed by skin scrubs or exfoliators.

The dermis contains two kinds of protein fibre, collagen and elastin, which give the skin the firmness and elasticity necessary to ensure it is tailor-made to fit each individual body and to expand and contract with the changing shape and size of that body. They also provide the resiliency required to cope with those everyday bumps and blows that we all experience. Collagen fibres, produced by special cells called fibroblasts, give the skin its strength and make up 75 percent of the dermis's weight. They are interwoven with the elastin fibres that make the skin stretchy. The gradual deterioration of these fibres is a result of the effect of our environment and the fact that their replacement rate drops off as we grow older. This is what makes the skin wrinkle and sag; the most obvious (and often dreaded) signs of ageing.

The skin provides a home to countless 'good' bacteria which defend our bodies against the threat of invasion from alien germs. When we take antibiotics, the skin's resident population of bacteria can be disturbed and our natural defences upset. This can result in itchy skin when you take some prescription drugs.

The Life Cycle of Our Skin

When we are born our skin contains plenty of moisture and has thick and strong, closely packed collagen fibres, making it look

WHAT IS ACNE?

smooth and supple, with invisible pores. At this stage the skin is thin and the sebaceous glands have not fully developed, which makes it very sensitive and prone to infection.

During childhood, the sebaceous glands develop and they are then activated by male hormones at puberty.

When we reach adolescence we experience a number of hormonal changes and these shift our now developed sebaceous glands into overdrive. They now produce a great deal of oil or sebum, making the skin appear oily and coarse. As a result of the overproduction of oil, adolescent skin is more prone to spots and blackheads than at any other time in the skin's life cycle. As we move through adulthood our skin starts to dry out naturally and the process is further accelerated by lifestyle factors such as exposure to the elements: wind, water, cold weather and sunshine.

Women who take the contraceptive pill usually find it has a drying effect on the skin because the oestrogen content reduces the activity of the sebaceous glands. This is why women who are on the pill often find their skin improves and they have less spots while they are taking it.

After the age of thirty our skin becomes thinner and its ability to repair itself slows down as the flow of blood to the lower regenerating layers is reduced. The production of sebum also slows down which adds to the drying out of the skin, making it thinner and more vulnerable to damage.

In middle age the lower dermal layer of skin loses its tone, causing the skin to become wrinkled and sag. A lifetime of exposure to the sun, in particular ultraviolet (UV) rays, is the main cause of skin ageing. Together with the slowing down of collagen and elastin production, stress, long-term exposure to the elements and lack of muscle tone all add to the effects. For women, skin ageing accelerates after the menopause when there is a noticeable loss of collagen, although to some extent this can be prevented by taking hormone replacement therapy (HRT).

Causes of Acne

Acne is the result of the skin reacting abnormally to levels of the male hormone testosterone in the blood, although the precise cause of this abnormal reaction is unknown. Testosterone activates the sebaceous glands at puberty in girls and boys and the glands start to produce oil to lubricate the skin. In sufferers of acne the level of sebum secretion is abnormally high because of the sensitivity of the sebaceous glands on different areas of the body, particularly on the face and the back, to testosterone.

The skin cells lining the hair ducts also react abnormally to testosterone and become sticky. Instead of dead cells being shed on to the surface of the skin, these accumulate in the duct and partially block it, obstructing the flow of sebum from the glands. The oil eventually solidifies and blocks the duct. The plug then becomes pigmented or coloured, resulting in the blackheads and whiteheads which are acne's non-inflammatory spots.

However, inflammation of the skin is also a symptom of acne. The inflammation and pus that forms in the skin of some acne sufferers is not really understood. It is thought that the partial blockage of the duct becomes a total blockage and the oil that has accumulated is broken down by bacteria. Inflammatory chemicals are then formed. The chemicals penetrate the skin and cause redness and swelling and the area becomes itchy and tender. Pus cells also form and the result of this process is that a pustule develops and eventually the pus ruptures on to the surface of the skin. If the inflammation is deep down in the hair duct or if the spot is squeezed before it is ready, then the pus may rupture beneath the skin's surface causing even more inflammation.

Who Gets Acne?

The tendency to develop acne is genetic, in the same way that having thick hair or brown eyes is, and, although we don't actually inherit spots, we can inherit a sensitivity to hormonal changes.

AGGRAVATING FACTORS
There is a range of other factors that affect acne. The debate still rages over the relationship between diet and acne. Most dermatologists agree that diet has no bearing on the cause of the condition and some would even say that acne is not made worse by eating the wrong foods. So, in theory, if you suffer from acne you can go ahead and indulge in pizza, chocolates, ice cream, fish and chips and fizzy drinks to your heart's content. However, this kind of diet is not going to do your heart or blood vessels any good.

Complementary practitioners take a different view. With their holistic approach to health problems, ie looking at a patient's problem as part of their whole being and not just a problem in itself, they believe that what you put inside your body is reflected on the outside. The quality of your diet is reflected in your skin tone – so if you eat a healthy diet your skin and body in general will be healthier as a result.

Whoever you choose to believe in the diet/acne debate, it is common sense that following a balanced diet including lots of fruit and vegetables is going to be beneficial to your health and general well-being, even if it has only a slight bearing on whether or not you get acne.

Grades and Types of Acne

You can take two people with acne and on one the condition may be barely noticeable, while on the other the skin may have

ACNE

been ravaged by acne to such an extent that there are numerous scars and cysts. This is because people have different amounts of acne and experience it in varying degrees of severity. Acne problems are generally divided into four grades:

Grade 1: *This level of acne means the skin is only affected by whiteheads and blackheads and they occur only on the face.*

Grade 2: *Here the skin looks oily; there are blackheads, whiteheads and pimples on the face and sometimes on the back and chest. This is the kind of acne that most teenagers suffer from at some time during adolescence and fortunately this type does not result in scarring (unless some of the spots are squeezed).*

Grade 3: *At this level the skin is very oily and, as well as the typical blackheads, whiteheads and pimples, there are also cysts which appear on the face, the back, neck and shoulders. Scarring can occur.*

Grade 4: *This form of acne has excessively oily skin, and sufferers have large cysts that overlap each other and make the skin raised in parts. Grade 4 acne appears on the same parts of the body as Grade 3 and frequently results in scarring.*

Not only does acne occur in varying degrees of severity, there are also a number of different kinds of acne. In theory all should disappear when we reach our twenties, when our hormone production settles down and we reach our full growth and sexual maturity. However, there are some types of acne that can affect adults at any time – not just the odd spot every month or so, but regular breakouts.

Acne can occur in adults as a result of not looking after the skin properly. This is obviously the most simple type to correct as it may just be a case of changing your skincare routine. Some of the cleansing creams on the market don't necessarily remove all the dirt and dead cells from our skin, and so they can leave it looking dull and can create the perfect environment for the

WHAT IS ACNE?

development of spots. Furthermore, moisturisers containing mineral oils are used in great quantities due to the widespread, and often irrational fear of having dry skin, and these can cause breakouts of blackheads, whiteheads and pimples. A change in routine can reduce acne and allow the skin to return to its normal, clear and healthy self. See Chapter 5 for steps to a clearer skin and tips on what we should be looking for when we choose our skincare products.

Dry skin acne is a relatively rare type which some adults suffer from. It sounds like a contradiction in terms, as people who suffer from acne usually have oily skin, but even very small amounts of oil can trigger acne problems in very sensitive people. Sometimes the problem may be due to the structure of the pore follicles – the size or shape of them can make it difficult for the oil to reach the skin's surface so it gets trapped and forms a whitehead.

A type of adult acne that has recently been referred to is 'career woman acne'. Dermatologist Dr Anthony Chu has observed a steady increase in the number of cases of career women who are suffering from acne. 'These are patients who sailed through their teens and twenties without any spots and now suddenly start to have problems.' Dr Chu is cautious about the reasons for this but does believe that stress is involved. 'Stress makes any skin condition much worse, so it wouldn't be surprising if the fact that these women are often in high-pressure jobs was a factor.' When we are stressed we all produce extra supplies of androgens (male hormones) which stimulate the oil glands into overdrive. Studies in the United States have shown that a fifth of women who have adult acne also have increased levels of these hormones in their blood. The acne appears on the cheeks, chin, neck and back and the blackheads tend to be quite pronounced. Dr Chu's comments are reaffirmed by research from a dermatological centre in southern California. This shows that post-adolescent acne is on the increase. Thirty percent of the

ACNE

patients at the dermatological centre are working, married and have children, a combination which can lead to significant stress.

ROSACEA PROBLEMS

Rosacea acne is a different kind of acne, but is still a fairly common problem, particularly in the middle-aged (which is why it is sometimes referred to as adult acne). The symptoms of this skin condition range from recurrent blushing attacks, to permanently red skin with broken veins or acne-like eruptions with lumps and pustules.

Approximately one in ten women between the ages of thirty and fifty-five suffer from some form of rosacea acne and, although it is not as common in men, those who do suffer tend to have a more severe form called rhinophyma, which affects the skin on the nose. This makes the skin thicken and turn a deep purple-red colour. The nose looks large and deformed and it can be wrongly assumed that the sufferer has a 'drinker's nose'. Eyelid irritations and other eye problems can also appear with rosacea.

Rosacea can be aggravated by certain aspects of our diet. Drinks that contain caffeine, such as tea, coffee and cola can all cause problems. So too can spicy foods. If you notice there is a correlation between what you eat and any changes in your condition, you should begin to eliminate aggravating foods from your diet and reduce your caffeine intake. (See Chapter 4 for tips on eating for a clearer skin.)

Stress is also a factor, although it can be more difficult to avoid than other triggers. If stress is a problem, try relaxation techniques like breathing exercises, yoga or meditation tapes.

In a study of rosacea acne conducted by the Acne Support Group, many sufferers found that certain types of food and drink affected the problem and, as a result, 56 percent of people with the skin condition avoided alcohol; 49 percent spicy foods; and 27 percent coffee. This survey also showed that rosacea acne had a damaging effect on the emotions and self-esteem of those affected by the condition. All who participated in the survey felt embarrassed and self-conscious about their condition, with a quarter believing it had a detrimental effect on long-term friendships and relationships. One-fifth believed it had a detrimental effect on sexual relationships and another fifth felt that their family life had been affected as a result of their condition and the effect it had on their confidence. Furthermore, one in six took time off work as a result of having rosacea and one in five believed it to be the cause of difficulties in gaining new employment or promotion.

It is important to see your GP if you think you may be suffering from rosacea as, unlike acne vulgaris, in most cases it is not a passing phase. As time goes by, the bouts of flushing become more frequent, more intense and longer lasting and the skin feels tender and swollen. The redness also becomes permanent. The face appears blotchy and may suddenly erupt into acne-like spots and bumps. Your GP will be able to prescribe antibiotics such as retronidazole gel or tetracycline tablets which are effective against rosacea acne. Severe or persistent cases should always be referred to an experienced dermatologist.

The Myths Surrounding Acne

To add insult to injury there are many myths and a great deal of misinformation surrounding this condition, which serves only to add to the confusion and suffering of those who are affected. Dr Anthony Chu also believes that it is 'one of the very few diseases in which sufferers are ridiculed because of their disease rather than offered sympathy', which is a result of the fact that 'society views acne as something to be laughed at and to be ashamed of'. Teenagers and children can be especially cruel with their teasing.

ACNE

The following statements dispel some of the common misunderstandings that surround the condition:

* Sexual habits do not play a role in teenage acne. Sexual activity has no bearing on acne and is definitely not the cause of it. The only link that exists between sex and acne is that, after puberty, the increase in production of male hormones, or androgens (which affect sexual development), also causes the increase of oil in the glands.
* Acne cannot be passed on through contact with a sufferer. Even though the spots are filled with pus, the germs that they contain, which are called saprophytes, are present on the skin at all times. If you have acne you simply have more of these. The germs are not contagious and you cannot get acne by being in close contact with someone who has it.
* Acne is not psychological in origin, although state of mind and other factors such as stress can certainly have a bearing on the condition. In reality acne is far more likely to be the cause of psychological traumas rather than a symptom, producing complexes in adolescents who are already self-conscious about their bodies and the way they look. In severe cases it can lead to a total loss of confidence, a distorted body image and lack of achievement in work, study and socially.
* Another myth is that acne is a teenage condition. Although it is most common in young people it develops in different ways in different people. It can appear for the first time in the mid-twenties, or start in adolescence and clear up after a few years (usually by the age of twenty-five). Other people can still have acne in their forties and fifties: 1 percent of men and 5 percent of women still have significant problems with

acne. If you are in your thirties, forties, fifties or even sixties and still have acne, you are definitely not alone.

* A commonly held belief is that sunbathing is one of the best treatments for acne. Although some people will see an improvement almost immediately after they have been in the sun, this is temporary. And, to make matters worse, a few weeks afterwards many people notice an increase in the number of whiteheads on their skin. When considering sunbathing as a method of treating acne it is also important to remember the damaging effects the sun, and particularly UV rays, have on the skin in the long term. When sunbathing use an adequate sun protection cream (dermatologists recommend a minimum of SPF15) and choose one that isn't oily. Sun lamps, often recommended to acne sufferers, also produce damaging UV rays.

2

Conventional Treatments for Acne

The good news about this potentially distressing skin condition is that it can be treated, and treated successfully – as long as the professional advice is followed and the treatment is used correctly. In this chapter we look at some of the conventional preparations used to treat acne that are available both over-the-counter (OTC) and on prescription. We also look at treatments like dermabrasion and cosmetic surgery as a response to scarring from acne.

One factor which is important to bear in mind is that acne does last for a long time, even with effective treatment. Approximately 80 percent of sufferers should see an 80 percent improvement in their skin within six months of treatment; however, this treatment may need to be continued for a period of years. Dr Nicholas Lowe, Clinical Professor of Dermatology at UCLA, says he usually sees excellent improvements within six – eight weeks with patients who are prescribed a combination of antibiotics and Retin-A.

Over-the-Counter Medication

A wide range of preparations are available from your pharmacist without a prescription, all of which are applied topically, ie directly to the skin. These include anti-bacterial skin washing creams, lotions and soaps which work on reducing the bacterial

ACNE

activity on the skin. Antiseptic creams, ointments and soap can destroy micro-organisms, and abrasives help to remove blockages that are clogging up the skin.

One of the most common forms of treatment for acne is benzoyl peroxide cream. Benzoyl peroxide is a powerful oxidising agent which peels skin, acts an anti-blackhead agent, reduces the amount of bacteria on the skin and reduces sebum production from the oil glands. A side-effect of this cream is that it can make the skin feel sore, but it is available in different strengths (2.5, 5 and 10 percent) to cater for this – if you have sensitive skin 2.5 percent should be used in the first instance and increased as your skin becomes more tolerant. Applying benzoyl peroxide for the first time will probably cause a burning sensation on your skin, and in the first few days the skin surface will redden and peel. If this continues for longer you should stop using the cream and consult your GP. Ask to be referred to a dermatologist, who will know more about up-to-date alternatives than a GP.

Some of the creams and lotions readily available from your local pharmacy include: Acnegel and cream, Boots Mediclear Acne Cream 5 and 10; Clearasil Medicated Cream, Cleansing Milk and Lotion; Oxy 5 and 10; Sudocrem; and TCP Antiseptic Liquid. Dermatologist Dr Nicholas Lowe suggests trying washing creams formulated with benzoyl peroxide in cases of early or mild acne. He also recommends certain preparations containing sodium lactate, such as Userin Plus.

Unfortunately OTC medications do not work for all acne sufferers and if you experience worrying side-effects or there appears to be no improvement in your skin, then you will need to see your GP or dermatologist who may prescribe a cream that contains retinoic acid or an antibiotic or anti-inflammatory cream. Antibiotics can also be prescribed for acne in both topical and tablet form.

CONVENTIONAL TREATMENTS FOR ACNE

Topical Antibiotics

Antibiotics have two functions: the first is to reduce the number of bacteria within the glands; the second is to reduce the inflammation of the skin.

The topical antibiotics used to treat acne include tetracycline, minocycline, erythromycin and clindamycin, which are all absorbed into the skin, reducing the level of bacteria and inflammation in the skin. They are prescribed for acne where there are pustules present, but they have no effect on blackheads. The side-effect of topical antibiotics is that the alcohol solutions they come in can irritate the skin and even dry it out. If this is a problem, clindamycin is available in a lotion form .

Oral Antibiotics

Oral antibiotics are usually prescribed for a minimum period of six months, either on their own, or in combination with topical treatments. The four groups that are commonly used are tetracyclines, erythromycin, trimethoprim and clindamycin. All groups work on reducing the number of bacteria on the skin as well as having an effect on inflammation within the skin.

Tetracyclines

These are the most effective antibiotics against acne. Unfortunately there are a number of side-effects. They can affect the contraceptive pill, making it unsafe and necessary to use an alternative form of contraceptive. They should not be prescribed to children under nine years of age as they can cause staining of the teeth. Tetracyclines can also cause thrush as a result of altering the microflora of the vagina. They should not be prescribed during pregnancy.

Erythromycin

This is relatively effective against inflammatory acne and has the bonus of having no effect on the contraceptive pill or on a developing foetus, so it is often prescribed to women of child-bearing age instead of tetracycline. Unfortunately it also can cause thrush.

Trimethoprim

This is effective in the treatment of acne and is generally a very safe drug. Occasionally it may cause nausea and a rare complication is the development of painful lumps on the legs.

Clindamycin

This is a very strong antibiotic which is used in severe cases of acne and is usually only prescribed when other antibiotics have failed. In rare cases it can cause diarrhoea. If you are taking clindamycin and this occurs, stop taking the tablets immediately and consult your GP.

Other Treatments

Retin-A

Retin-A comes in a gel cream or lotion form and is available in 0.025 percent (the mildest) and 0.05 percent (one of the strongest) concentrations.

A derivative of vitamin A, Retin-A (also called tretinoin) affects the development of the skin cells, so it is used when the hair canal is blocked. It literally forces out the oil and the skin cells that have accumulated. It is effective against blackheads by softening the skin and making the blackheads literally drop off. Unfortunately, in many cases, Retin-A is very irritating to the skin and not only causes soreness and redness, but in some people can even crack the skin. It should be used in the lowest

CONVENTIONAL TREATMENTS FOR ACNE

dosage to begin with so that the skin can build up in order to cleanse itself. It is not generally considered suitable for those with a combination of acne and eczema. However, many people achieve excellent results with Retin-A – its beneficial side-effects include reducing wrinkles! However, it can cause a permanent sensitivity to the sun, requiring a life-long use of sun protection creams.

Dianette

Dianette is a brand of contraceptive pill that contains a medium dose of oestrogen and also a drug called cyproterone acetate that counters the effect of testosterone and reduces the production of grease. It is only suitable for treating women who have acne, and can be effective where other therapies have failed. Many women find that their skin clears when on any form of the contraceptive pill as the oestrogen content reduces the activity of the sebaceous glands.

At the start of treatment with Dianette it is common for acne to flare up; however, as treatment progresses it settles down. A side-effect, as with other forms of hormonal treatment, can be depression, and some women also experience stomach upsets.

Isotretinoin

Isotretinoin is a synthetic form of vitamin A that can only be prescribed by a hospital dermatologist. It is used to treat people suffering from severe cystic acne that hasn't responded to antibiotics. Isotretinoin has been described as revolutionising the treatment of acne, even in those who are severely affected – and it works on both inflammatory and non-inflammatory blackheads. The effects are dramatic and when treatment ends the skin is usually clear and the acne does not recur to the same extent.

Unfortunately, everyone who takes isotretinoin develops sore chapped lips and most also have dry itchy skin. Many people also experience joint or muscle pains, and recurrent nasal bleeding and dryness. Furthermore, the drug can also affect the liver and the amount of fat in the blood, requiring blood tests before a course is started. When the drug is prescribed to women of childbearing age, the use of an effective contraceptive (usually meaning the oral contraceptive) is compulsory, as the drug is unsafe for unborn babies.

NEW TREATMENTS

A prescription-only product for the topical treatment of acne, which has only recently become available in this country, is a combination of two tried and tested substances that are used in the treatment of acne: benzoyl peroxide and erythromycin. The claim is that the 'synergistic action' between these two components makes this treatment fast acting and effective. The benzoyl peroxide unblocks sebaceous glands, reducing the number of blackheads, and erythromycin has an antibacterial effect, inhibiting the production of a vital bacterial enzyme.

The product, produced by Bioglan Laboratories, has been endorsed by Dr Anthony Chu, who believes that it 'offers advantages to acne patients, particularly the short time between starting the therapy and seeing an improvement in the condition of the skin, which motivates them to use the product regularly'. Dr Chu is in the process of carrying out his own tests on the effect of the cream on those suffering from moderate to severe acne. The results of this test are not available at the time of writing.

Guidelines to Using Acne Treatments

As we have seen, there is a wide range of available treatments effective in the battle against acne. However, it is important to remember that it will be a long battle. Acne is slow to respond

CONVENTIONAL TREATMENTS FOR ACNE

and there may be little or no improvement in the first month of treatment. After two months you may see up to a 40 percent improvement and by the end of six months this should have doubled. It is important to seek medical help as soon as acne occurs, and remember that it requires continuous treatment. If your child has acne, do not wait until it takes hold and scars the skin – seek assistance without delay.

TABLETS

The antibiotics tetracycline and erythromycin are usually taken twice a day. These should be taken approximately half an hour before eating, with water. If you forget to take the tablet *before* you eat a meal, don't wait until the next meal – take it straight away. If you have been prescribed doxycycline, minocycline, trimethoprim or isotretinoin, these should be taken *after* you have eaten.

Most acne sufferers will not have to take tablets for the rest of their lives and if the acne responds well to treatment, it may be possible to give up the tablets gradually and switch to using a topical cream or lotion. A few spots may recur when you stop a course of antibiotics, although applying cream continuously should reduce the risk of this problem.

CREAMS, GELS AND LOTIONS

General guidelines are to apply the treatment twice a day (although this does differ with certain creams and gels and there will be instructions in the packet – if you have any queries check with your GP or pharmacist). Apply to the whole area of skin affected by acne, not just to the spots individually, as this helps to prevent new spots from developing.

Some creams that are designed to treat acne can cause redness and scaling. If you have a severe response to a particular cream or lotion, stop the treatment altogether for a couple of days, then start to reapply to one area at a time. If there is a problem with your neck, for example, try using the cream just on your back and then gradually reintroduce it to areas of skin that are affected by acne. If irritation recurs, follow this procedure again. Unfortunately it seems to be the case that some of the most effective topical treatments for acne result in a certain amount of redness and scaling. Using a hypo-allergenic moisturising cream may help relieve the dryness and irritation.

Don't forget that some treatments, particularly those which contain benzoyl peroxide (a bleaching agent) have to be allowed to dry on your skin before you get dressed or go to bed, otherwise you could end up with tie-dyed sheets and pillows or clothing.

Acne Scars

Sufferers of severe acne may develop scarring. If scarring is minimal most people find that they can live with it and that it does improve over time. However, if scarring is extensive, there are some surgical measures that can be considered. Acne can cause both pitted and thick, raised (or keloid) scarring.

PITTED SCARRING
Pitted scarring is the result of inflammation in the skin and pus formation which has actually damaged the structural component of the skin and, as with injuries like cuts and abscesses, the body heals the damage with scar tissue. This type of scarring is so called because the skin looks like it has pits in it or it has a dented effect. Pitted scars can either be large and crater-like with well-defined edges, or small, as if someone has pushed a spike into the skin (commonly referred to as ice pick scars). Unfortunately, as acne can affect large sections of the skin, the scarring can also be spread over a large area. Although it is permanent, there may be some improvement with time.

CONVENTIONAL TREATMENTS FOR ACNE

The bottom line is that once pitted scarring has occurred, the skin is never going to be perfect again. However, there is some good news – there are a number of cosmetic procedures that can improve the skin's appearance. The main aim, however, should be to prevent scarring before it occurs with the aid of the active treatments described at the beginning of this chapter. Professor Lowe suggests a trip to the doctor if the acne is itching so much that the temptation to scratch is very great. He treats cases of 'itchers' with prompt applications of an antibiotic cream or cortisone injections to avoid self-inflicted scarring.

Dermabrasion

This operation is usually carried out under general anaesthetic by plastic surgeons and the success rate is between 20 and 60 percent (depressed scars respond better than the ice pick variety). A high speed wire brush or diamond burr is used to literally plane off the top layers of skin. Obviously the skin will feel pretty sore afterwards and the area that has been treated will form a scab which should fall away after a week. This should reveal smoother, underlying skin. However, in some cases, dermabrasion can actually make the skin look worse, so it is important to discuss both your individual problem and the operation thoroughly with your dermatologist and the plastic surgeon, and to be prepared for the possibility of this outcome. Many surgeons perform a small test area of dermabrasion under local anaesthetic to project the results, before undertaking treatment on the whole area. There are a number of hospitals that offer dermabrasion on the NHS, but the wait tends to be quite long. To have the treatment carried out privately costs somewhere in the region of £1,500. Always check to ensure that the cosmetic surgeon performing the operation is very experienced.

ACNE

Chemical peeling

With this form of treatment, a chemical is applied to the skin which burns it and then lifts off the top layer. Phenol is the most widely used substance in this country. This procedure is only beneficial for skin that has mild, superficial scarring and has little effect on deep scarring.

Check with your GP for availability on the NHS in your area. Treated privately you could expect to pay anywhere between £1,000 and £2,000. Again, it is very important to ensure that the cosmetic surgeon you consult is highly experienced with skin peeling procedures.

Collagen injections

The purified collagen from cow skin is injected into the living layer of the epidermis in areas where there is scarring. This adds to the skin's natural collagen, filling the dents in the skin. This works most effectively on soft pitted scars, although scars with defined edges and ice pick scars do not normally respond to this form of treatment.

In some cases collagen can cause an allergic reaction (only around 1 percent of patients are usually affected) so a test dose is injected into the arm to check for a reaction. Unfortunately, improvement with collagen injections is not permanent and although they can be topped up every twelve–twenty-four months, they're not cheap! Expect to pay £360 for treatment comprising six syringe injections of 0.5ml of collagen, plus £20 for the initial skin test, plus the cost of a consultation with the physician and his or her time and skill in injecting the collagen. Check with your GP for availability on the NHS in your area.

KELOID SCARRING

Keloid scars are the raised lumpy kind that can result from any kind of acne although some people's skin is naturally more likely to respond to acne in this way than others'. In the skin an

CONVENTIONAL TREATMENTS FOR ACNE

abnormal healing process takes place and the production of scar tissue becomes exaggerated. The scars grow slowly in size, have a smooth surface and can be round or oblong. Keloid scars respond best to treatment when they are still active, ie tender or itchy. Keloids that are established do not respond well (sometimes not at all) to treatment.

Treatment

Keloid scars are not only disfiguring; they can also be painful and itchy. Treatment is required as soon as possible after they have formed – the earlier the treatment the better the response. Treatment will flatten keloid scars and the pain and itchiness will disappear but, unfortunately, the skin will never return to normal.

* *Steroid injections.* Steroid solutions can be injected directly into the keloids. Although a local anaesthetic is used, this is still a painful procedure. The process needs to be repeated every four to six weeks. The earlier this treatment is started, the better the results – although response rates do vary. If the response is good, the lumpy characteristic of keloid scarring will disappear along with any pain and itchiness. The scar will be flattened and there will be a remaining area of discolouration.
* *Steroid creams.* Steroid creams can help to flatten keloids. The results are not as good as with steroid injections and if they are used for a long period of time the skin surrounding the keloid scar can become thin and broken blood vessels may develop in this area.
* *Surgery.* In most cases keloid scars cannot be removed by surgery – if surgery is performed, the wound simply develops into an even larger keloid scar. In rare cases, keloids can be removed from the skin and the site of the wound treated with radiotherapy in order to

prevent the keloid scar re-forming. This is not always successful but may be an option if conventional therapy does not work.

Acne Sufferers and Their GPs

There has been some criticism of the attitude that GPs have towards patients suffering from acne. Many patients have found, when requesting advice, that the response they get is often far from sympathetic. Dr Colin Clark, himself a GP based in Glasgow, says that 'Acne continues to be regarded as a low priority condition by GPs who often dismiss it as trivial and something which will right itself.' He believes that 'patients who have been inadequately treated on conventional acne treatments would have less scarring if they had been referred for early oral isotretinoin treatment. Indeed, the best treatment for acne scars is to prevent them and isotretinoin treatment has been proved to be less expensive than long courses of often ineffective antibiotics. GPs should send patients to dermatologists earlier.'

In his book *New Approaches to Acne Treatment* (Martin Dunitz Ltd. 1994), which is a guide for the medical profession, Dr W J Cunliffe recommends that GPs follow these principles in the treatment of acne sufferers:

* Consider acne as a physical and psychological disease
* Treat acne as a serious disease
* Remember that acne is a very treatable disease
* Treat the patient with enthusiasm
* Refer the patient to a dermatologist if their response is less than ideal
* Treat sooner rather than later to prevent any scarring
* Consider oral isotretinoin sooner rather than later.

CONVENTIONAL TREATMENTS FOR ACNE

The hope then, is that GPs will become more aware of the problems that acne sufferers experience and will treat them with sensitivity. The general consensus of opinion regarding treatment for acne seems to be that sufferers of severe acne should be referred to a dermatologist. If your GP is not forthcoming in recommending this avenue of treatment, do suggest you are being referred to a dermatologist, as, unless you go privately, the referral has to come from your GP.

3

A Natural Approach

The pimples that are characteristic of acne, whether they are red lumps, yellow pustules or blackheads, are all teeming with bacteria, so the main form of conventional treatment is with high doses of antibiotics. But, as we have seen in the previous chapter, these are not without side-effects, such as thrush in women.

Furthermore, resistance to the antibiotics can also develop, especially when the antibiotics are prescribed over a period of months. This can leave the body open to more serious infections. For this reason, many people choose to take a natural approach to treating acne.

A vital function of the skin is that it is one of the body's main organs of elimination. Many complementary practitioners believe acne to be a sign of an imbalance in the system with eruptions on the skin the result of the body failing to eliminate its toxins and waste effectively. So in the first instance it is important to help the body cleanse itself.

We sweat approximately one pint of liquid on a daily basis (without taking into account any vigorous activity). The sweat is not simply made up of water, but contains salt, potassium and waste in the form of uric acid, urea (both from chemical breakdown of protein) ammonia and lactic acid. If for some reason the body's organs are not working to their full potential, ie you're constipated or your kidneys have been working overtime, then more of the body's waste is expelled through the skin resulting in a dull complexion and skin problems. So, even though there is no proven link between acne and a bad diet, if you do have acne, it makes things easier on your skin if you follow a diet that:

* nourishes the skin
* helps with any elimination problems your body may be having
* ensures that the other organs of elimination are in top condition so you don't place any extra pressure on the skin

There are plenty of foods we can eat which actively encourage the elimination of waste from the body. But first the bad news: certain foods should be avoided in order to facilitate the eliminating process, as they are the ones which produce the most waste and toxins in the skin cells. These include milk, cream, sugar, processed foods and those containing many additives.

Homeostasis

The human body is like a wonderful self-generating machine. It heals and regulates itself through a process known as homeostasis. One of the key functions of homeostasis is to detoxify your body and this involves a number of bodily organs including the skin. The efficiency of these organs depends both on inherited factors and on how we treat our body. Some people seem to endlessly abuse their bodies and yet come out unscathed, while others are unable to cope with small levels of toxins and stress. This factor is probably genetic. However, it is possible to improve your levels of homeostasis.

THE BOWEL
The bowel shifts large amounts of waste daily but it can easily get clogged up due to a poor diet. If you think that one bowel

movement a day is good, then think again! Four-fifths of the food which you eat should be eliminated via the bowels and one bowel movement is probably not going to do the job.

Some of the food in our diet gets left behind in the colon causing a build-up of waste. Highly refined starches (such as cakes), dairy produce, eggs, sugar, prescription drugs and a lack of fluid and fibre are the main culprits. To maintain a healthy bowel, it is important to cut down on these foods and eat foods rich in fibre. Cutting down on wheat and other grains that contain gluten may also help to keep your bowels and colon clear.

INTESTINES

The food we eat passes from the stomach into the intestines where nutrients are absorbed and the residue is readied for elimination. This process involves about 400 different species of micro-organisms, some of which are necessary and some of which are not. Some of the good ones are *Bifido-bacteria* and *Lactobacillus acidophilus* (this is also found in live yoghurt), and these are superb agents of detoxification. They help to digest the food we have eaten as well as stimulating the peristaltic action (the movement which pushes the bowel contents along). If you suffer with constipation and sluggish intestines, don't overload your body and eat only when you feel hungry. Make sure you are eating a large amount of fruit, vegetables and whole grains to get all the fibre you need. Eating dried fruits like figs and prunes regularly should get things moving. It is also extremely important to keep fluid intake high, so aim to drink at least 1.5 litres of pure water daily (in addition to hot drinks).

KIDNEYS

The action of the kidneys is twofold. They eliminate toxins from the blood through urine and they also salvage and re-absorb valuable nutrients which can be recycled for future use by the body. Our bodies are filled mainly with water and we eliminate about four and a half litres of water every day through the skin, the kidneys and the other organs of elimination. Unfortunately, the efficiency of this filter effect diminishes with age or excessive toxicity due to diet, drugs or a toxic environment. If your kidneys are not working to their full capacity it will be apparent in your urine (it may be strong smelling, darkly coloured or cloudy). Eating fennel, leeks, onions and raw cabbage will help your kidneys to work more efficiently. Or try drinking an infusion of nettle tea. Asparagus juice is a particularly good kidney cleanser, and increasing your intake of pure water works well too.

LIVER

This important organ of detoxification has over 1,500 different functions, from secreting bile to the formation of blood. It processes all foods (except for some fats) which have been absorbed by the intestines, before releasing the nutrients into the bloodstream. The liver also filters the blood, removing, deactivating or reprocessing toxins, wastes and bacteria, but if it is bombarded with too many toxins, its ability to detox will be diminished. If your liver is functioning below par you may feel nauseous, have indigestion or a furry tongue. Eating grapes, celery, apples, carrots, olives/olive oil and drinking dandelion tea will all help it to work more effectively. Silymarin (milk thistle) supplements can also be taken to strengthen liver functioning.

LUNGS

Any toxic debris left in your internal system can be exhaled through the lungs. In fact, far more is passed this way than through urine. Our lungs are constantly flushing out carbon dioxide and carbonic acid wastes every time we breathe out. Unfortunately, toxic pollutants which are inhaled reach the bloodstream more quickly than those arriving via the digestive system as less filtering is performed by the lungs. It is important always to breathe in through the nose and breathe out through the mouth to keep clearing the lungs of toxins. One of the best expectorants to clear the lungs is garlic, preferably fresh, although you can buy garlic capsules in health food shops.

LYMPHATICS

Lymph is a fluid derived from the blood and it is carried around the body via a vast network of vessels. The lymphatic drainage system, interacting with the bloodstream through special ducts, depends mainly on the pump action of breathing and the action of our muscles as they contract and expand during use. Lymph vessels contain a huge amount of white blood cells which attack invaders and clean out waste matter. These key immune function agents are called lymphocytes and macrophages and they protect us against infection, cancer and toxicity. Lymph passes through a series of filters (lymph nodes), found in the neck, armpits, groin and backs of the knees. The lymphatic drainage system plays an important part in the removal of waste, but it can easily become clogged up by a diet which is too rich in foods that the body finds difficult to deal with, such as red meat, dairy produce, sugar, fried food and synthetic substances.

SKIN

The skin is an extremely efficient back-up for the other organs of elimination. The hundreds of thousands of sweat glands in the skin act like mini-kidneys, detoxifying other organs and cleansing the blood. In order for the skin to carry out this important job effectively, the pores of the skin need to be unblocked. Signs of elimination problems become visible in the form of spots, blotches, boils, etc. One of the best ways to remove the dead skin cells which often block the skin pores is to use a body brush. A brush made from natural fibres with a wooden base and detachable long wooden handle is needed for

ACNE

skin brushing. You should start to brush upwards from your feet to your hips and always brush in the direction of your heart. When brushing your back, brush upwards from your bottom towards the middle of your back and then brush downwards over each shoulder. Skin brushing not only removes dirt and dead skin from the stratum corneum (outer layer of skin), but it also boosts circulation and lymphatic drainage which will help to eliminate waste internally. Do this daily, prior to bathing or showering.

Exercising regularly will also help, as exercise increases the blood flow to the surface of the skin, improving the process of nourishing the skin cells and carrying away waste matter.

Herbal Healing

Herbs have been used in the treatment and prevention of illness for thousands of years and at one time, from Rome and Greece to China and Russia, they formed the basis of all medicine. There are many herbs that can improve the condition of the skin and help to control acne. Some can be applied to the skin directly in the form of washes and creams as well as being taken internally as tonics. You only have to look as far as your fridge or vegetable rack for many effective natural remedies.

ALOE VERA GEL

The aloe plant originates from tropical Africa and was used to treat wounds from poisoned arrows. It was also used widely by the Greeks and Romans for treating wounds. The gel is useful for a range of skin conditions and helps to get rid of pimples. Massage aloe vera gel into the skin in the morning and at night as it also helps treat the scarring that can be caused by acne. Some skin tonics also contain aloe vera and are worth trying.

A NATURAL APPROACH

BURDOCK
Particularly valuable for the effective functioning of the liver and kidneys, burdock also helps to clear the skin. Boil the root in a cupful of water and leave to infuse for ten minutes. Drink three times a day.

CABBAGE
Cabbage has anti-bacterial and anti-inflammatory properties and is both nutritious and healing. Make a skin lotion by liquidising 250g of fresh leaves with 250ml of witchhazel, strain, then add two drops of lemon oil.

CALENDULA
Calendula (the marigold flower) acts as a herbal astringent, antiseptic and a natural anti-inflammatory. Mix a teaspoon of tincture of calendula (you can buy the tincture from health food stores) in a glass of water, strain as necessary then bathe the affected area with the lotion using cotton wool.

CHAMOMILE
Chamomile has relaxant and anti-inflammatory properties. Put a teaspoon of dried camomile flowers, or even a chamomile tea bag, in a cup of boiled water and then cover the cup and leave to infuse for ten minutes. Use the liquid as a face wash or skin tonic.

DANDELION
This grows in abundance all over the countryside. Pick the young fresh leaves and add them to a green salad or make into a vegetable soup. The herb is one of the best natural cleansers, detoxifiers and tonics available. Dandelion tea and coffee is available from health food shops.

ACNE

ECHINACEA

Echinacea, also known as the purple coneflower, originates from the northern USA and is now cultivated in Europe. It was used by native Americans to treat snakebite, fevers and non-healing wounds. Early settlers also adopted it as a remedy for colds and flu. Echinacea has been valued for centuries as an antiseptic and system purifier, but recently researchers have also been investigating the herb's usefulness as an immuno-stimulant – helping the body fight bacterial and viral infections (it has even been used in AIDS therapy).

Echinacea has also attracted much interest recently as a herbal treatment for a variety of skin conditions including eczema, psoriasis and acne. It contains active ingredients which help to form fibroblasts (the cells that develop into connective tissue) and it also boosts the skin's natural healing processes. Numerous studies have confirmed that echinacea helps to form healthy, new skin and it can be taken both internally and applied topically to the skin.

Potters Herbal Suppliers have a range of products called Skin Clear which have been developed to treat spots, pimples and mild acne and the tablets from the range contain echinacea. These are available from health food shops. Echinacea ointment is also helpful for acne sufferers as it helps to eliminate any dirt particles on the skin, so as to avoid secondary skin infections. It also helps to relieve pain, promote the formation of epidermal skin and avoid scarring. Some high-quality skincare products contain echinacea extract so look out for these.

FENNEL

This is one of the many herbs which act as diuretics, helping to flush out toxins in increased production of urine. Fennel also stimulates the circulation. It tastes of aniseed and the fresh bulb can be chopped and added to salads, while a delicious herbal tea can be bought from health food shops.

Garlic

Garlic is a quick and simple way of treating acne. It has antibacterial and antifungal properties, which have an effective antiseptic action on infected skin conditions. Simply cut a clove of garlic in half and rub on the affected area. It's a good idea to do this at night, as garlic isn't everyone's favourite fragrance. If you can't face putting garlic on your skin make sure you use plenty in your cooking or take a daily garlic supplement. Many deodorised forms are available in either tablet or capsule form which have all the beneficial properties but won't be detected on your breath!

Lavender

Lavender is a powerful herbal antiseptic which helps to promote healing. Place a handful of lavender flowers in a bowl with boiling water and give yourself a facial steam. Sit with your face at a comfortable distance from the steaming water and cover both your head and the bowl with a towel. Never steam your face for more than fifteen minutes and stop as soon as it starts to feel uncomfortable.

Rosemary

This culinary herb stimulates circulation and it has a relaxing and restorative effect on the nervous system. It is also highly antiseptic and a few drops of rosemary essential oil added to a warm bath make a soothing anti-bacterial soak, which is especially useful in cases of acne on the back and chest.

Aromatherapy and Acne

Aromatherapy is the practice of using essential oils to produce a number of therapeutic responses. The oils are often used to massage the body where they act on olfactory nerves in the nose,

ACNE

and minute quantities are absorbed through the skin. Aromatherapists were revered in ancient Egypt but the modern practice of aromatherapy was developed in France by Madame Maury and Dr Jean Valnet in the 1920s. The essential oils can be blended with a base or carrier oil such as almond or grapeseed oil and massaged into the skin or, alternatively, a few drops of the oil can be added to water in the bath or sink. Each oil has a variety of properties, although the majority are antiseptic. Essential oils are very powerful in their undiluted form and they must be handled with care. Never add more than ten drops of essential oil to bath water and, when mixing them with a carrier oil, you should add one drop of the essential oil to every millilitre (ml) of carrier oil, ie five drops of oil for every 5ml, ten drops for every 10ml and so on. It is useful to know that 5ml = 1 teaspoon, 10ml = 1 dessertspoon and 15ml = 1 tablespoon. Do not add more than thirty drops of essential oil to the base oil as essential oils are very potent and can harm the skin. Only lavender and tea tree oils can be applied neat.

CHAMOMILE

Chamomile oil has antiseptic properties and soothes the inflammation caused by acne. Add two drops of the essential oil to a teaspoon of soya or peach kernel oil and apply to the face. Some facial creams and skin tonics contain chamomile extracts. A few drops of the concentrated essential oil may also be used in the bath – the more expensive German chamomile has a greater potency.

JUNIPER

The oil from juniper berries has been used traditionally to treat problem skin and a few drops can be used in facial oils for treating acne. It is also used as a detoxifier and is sometimes found in massage oils to treat cellulite and other skin conditions.

LAVENDER

Lavender essential oil is a very useful antiseptic healer. Use tiny dabs of neat lavender essential oil on spots and pustules. Avoid the eyes and lips and apply in small amounts using a cotton bud. The oil can also be diluted with wheatgerm oil and applied to dried spots to help prevent scarring. As it soothes pain, it is a useful item in the first-aid box. Lavender oil is one of the few essential oils that can be applied to the skin undiluted in small quantities.

Recipe suggestion: mix two drops each of juniper and lavender oil with approximately half a glass of water and bathe the affected areas of skin with the lotion.

MYRRH

Myrrh, used in religious ceremonies since time immemorial and by the ancient Egyptians for embalming purposes, has good antiseptic properties and also helps to reduce inflammation, so it's an effective oil for treating skin problems like acne. Add two to four drops of myrrh to a carrier oil such as soya, grapeseed or almond, then apply to the skin with cotton wool.

PATCHOULI

Patchouli comes from the dried branches of a plant that originates in Malaysia and the Seychelles. The oil is often used in perfumes, but it is also a good antiseptic and can be applied wherever there is infection. Patchouli helps to reduce inflammation so is helpful in treating acne as well as dermatitis and allergic reactions. Add two drops to two teaspoons of almond oil and rub on to the skin.

SANDALWOOD

This traditional Indian extract can be added to massage blends to treat sore, inflamed skin conditions such as acne. It is also good for sensitive skin conditions.

TEA TREE OIL

This comes from the leaves of the medicinal tea tree which grows in Australia. Aborigines have long been aware of this oil's incredible healing powers and used it to treat cuts, wounds and all manner of skin infections. They crushed tea tree leaves, placed them over the area of injury and then covered the area with warm mud.

Tea tree essential oil is particularly effective in treating acne, among other things, as it is a very powerful antiseptic, but at the same time it is also soothing and doesn't damage or aggravate sensitive skin. An Australian study which set out to discover the skin's tolerance to tea tree oil and its effect on acne compared with benzoyl peroxide showed that at 5 percent strength both reduced the number of pimples and, although tea tree oil was slower to work, it caused fewer side-effects than benzoyl peroxide. The oil can be applied directly on to spots with cotton wool or a cotton bud to help prevent infection. Test the oil on one pimple to begin with, in case of sensitivity.

Homoeopathy

Homoeopathic treatment is based on the principle that a substance which, in large doses, will cause the symptoms of an illness can be used in minute doses to relieve the same symptoms. The principle is often described as curing 'like with like'. In homoeopathic medicine there is great emphasis on the individuality of the patient so a full consultation with a practitioner is valuable. However, there are an increasing number of OTC remedies available which you can use to treat your symptoms. The following is a brief remedy finder.

ACNE VULGARIS
The choice of homoeopathic remedy depends on the type of acne.

A NATURAL APPROACH

* If acne is characterised by a tendency to form pus, use hepar sulphuris 6c in the first instance. If acne is characterised by a tendency to form pus, use hepar sulphuris 6c.
* If there are painful spots which never come to a head, use calcium sulphuris 6c.
* For chronic acne take kali bichromicum 6c and for acne that is so severe that it is likely to cause scarring try silica 6c.
* Psorinium 6c is recommended for severe and itchy infections.

ACNE ROSACEA

The following homoeopathic remedies should be taken up to three times daily for up to three weeks.

* If the face feels dry, and there is a burning sensation and the skin is flaky and scaly, try the remedy arsenicum 6c.
* In the early stages of acne rosacea, when the face is red, dry and hot, use belladonna 6c.
* For burning and itching that is aggravated by heat, the remedy sanguinaria 6c can be used.
* If acne rosacea is aggravated by alcohol, tea and coffee and if there is also irritability and constipation, use rhus toxicodendron 6c.
* For itchy painful spots and a puffy swollen face, try rhus toxicodendron 6c.
* If the symptoms of acne rosacea are worse in the morning and if the face is mottled and a reddish purple colour, try lachesis 6c.

Remedies are available from good health food stores, chemists and by mail order – see Useful Addresses. In most cases it is beneficial to have a consultation with a qualified homoeopath who will take a holistic approach to your health, looking at your diet, lifestyle and medical history to see which are the most appropriate treatments for you.

New Treatments

One of the newest and probably most unconventional forms of treatment for acne comes in the shape of a bitter green juice extracted from sharks. There have been claims from Japan that an extract of shark bile taken from the animal's gall bladder is effective against spots. However, some may feel that the idea of using shark bile to reduce their acne cruel, despite the fact that sharks are not an endangered species.

Tests conducted by Dr David Fenton, a dermatologist at St Thomas's Hospital in London, on fifteen patients using the juice as a spray, showed marked improvements in their acne, and on ceasing treatment, the acne returned. The shark bile treatment has been developed by a laboratory in Australia where it has been refined for human usage and labelled as Ket Sugo. Dr Fenton believes it may have an effect on acne by reducing the production of grease or natural sebum in the skin, but precisely how it works has yet to be determined.

4

The Anti-Acne Diet

Our skin reflects externally what's going on internally. In general, when we're healthy our complexion looks fresh and clear; if we are unhealthy or under stress it becomes ashen and sallow. Eating a varied and balanced diet, eliminating processed foods and saturated fats and having an active lifestyle is the key to looking and feeling good. This optimum lifestyle also helps to combat the potentially destructive psychological effects of chronic skin disorders.

As we have already suggested, there is no medical evidence to prove that a poor diet alone causes acne. This traditional medical view about the role of diet has been challenged by herbalists and alternative practitioners. Herbalist Annemarie Colbin, who practises in the USA, says that in her experience '... diet has everything to do with acne. Not only did I fix my own bad skin through eating correctly, but I have seen among my students a number of severe cases where the large purplish kind of acne on cheeks and chins was completely cured in three months by a change of diet.'

The diet/acne debate is ongoing but what is clear is that the treatment of acne and other chronic skin problems should go hand in hand with a balanced diet and a healthy lifestyle which includes taking regular exercise and reducing stress. Among other things, a diet high in saturated fats and lacking in essential nutrients can hinder the skin's healing processes and could even reduce the effectiveness of medical treatments.

Exercise and Our Skin

Taking regular exercise, particularly outdoors, is essential for clear and healthy skin. Good circulation ensures that a steady supply of oxygen-rich blood cells repairs, nourishes and builds new skin tissues. Plenty of exercise also keeps us looking young by strengthening the collagen and elastin structures in the dermis. Exercising outdoors also exposes the skin to daylight, so stimulating the production of vitamin D, which is thought to activate the healing of skin tissue. Remember to take care in the summer months and wear a cream with a high SPF (sun protection factor) to protect against the burning UV rays which damage the skin and aggravate existing skin problems.

The Stress Factor

Improving our general health also means reducing the amount of stress in our lives. The skin and the nervous system are closely related, so it's no coincidence that, in the first instance, acne usually occurs during the teenage years – a stressful and emotionally turbulent time. High levels of stress may also propel the sufferer towards bad habits which not only jeopardise the condition of the skin, but could also contribute to the development of skin disorders. Dependency on alcohol, cigarettes and caffeine are often an inherent part of a stressful lifestyle, as is the consumption of 'comfort foods' such as chocolate, sweets and highly processed junk foods.

'Trigger' Foods

Acne-prone skin can be affected by diet in various ways and a common complaint is that certain foods irritate and inflame

THE ANTI-ACNE DIET

affected areas. The so-called 'trigger' foods most commonly listed are spicy foods, foods with a high iodine content, such as seafood and kelp, foods containing high levels of fat and those that are packed with artificial additives. An allergic reaction to food causes the blood vessels to dilate and weaken, leading to skin inflammation and irritation. Sufferers of acne rosacea may be particularly sensitive to foods of differing extremes, such as hot spicy food and cold food such as ice-cream. Additionally, eating foods that are high in iodine can cause an excretion via the sebaceous glands which irritates sensitive skin, while an excess of chocolate, milk and refined sugars stimulates the production of sebum and may weaken the immune system.

Another group of foods to be avoided is saturated fats. These are the hard fats found in animal produce, such as fatty meat, lard and cheese. Saturated fats are one of the main causes of heart disease, which is annually responsible for 40 percent of all deaths in the U.K. Less chronic but still important, a high cholesterol intake also affects the health of our skin. Saturated fats clog up the arteries and block the lymphatic system which clears the body's waste materials. Increased levels of toxicity in the body lead to more waste matter being passed through the skin which ultimately results in fresh outbreaks of spots and pimples.

The answer is relatively simple: as far as possible avoid foods which can irritate and intensify acne.

FOODS TO AVOID

* Fatty foods such as crisps, fried foods, red meat, butter, lard.
* Foods with a high sugar content such as sweets and chocolates.
* Spicy foods.
* Highly processed convenience foods which contain additives.

ACNE

- ✱ Excessively iodised salt and foods with a high iodine content such as seafood – clams, shrimps, haddock, salmon, sardines and tuna fish.
- ✱ Alcohol and hot beverages.

Essential Nutrients

Further evidence of the links between diet and skin are the flare-ups and rashes that often occur when the body becomes deficient in essential nutrients and trace elements. A diet lacking in vitamins A (in the form of beta-carotene) and C has a major impact on the health and vitality of the skin. These vitamins work to repair damaged skin tissue and both are powerful antioxidants, which means they prevent the formation of destructive free radicals – substances that are produced by the body during the course of normal cell activity, but which in large quantities destroy the cells and fibrous proteins found in the skin. Nevertheless, free radicals are important in helping to rid the body of the waste products that build up as a result of the normal metabolic processes. If the body's cleansing system becomes sluggish, more waste and debris gets clogged up in the dermis and epidermis, and this can eventually encourage acne.

Zinc is an essential trace element and 20 percent of the body's zinc content is concentrated in the skin. Deficiency in this element is another important factor which may ultimately exacerbate skin disorders. Low levels of zinc in the body have been identified as contributing to the development of teenage acne. Some nutritionists recommend taking vitamin A and zinc supplements to anyone with acne.

Looking good is not high up on the body's agenda, and if there's a shortage of nutrients the critical areas are supplied first and the skin gets the leftovers. The effects of an unbalanced diet don't always show on the skin immediately, but over a period of time the skin will deteriorate in condition both on the surface and in the dermal tissues. The complex structural make-up of the skin, the diversity of its functions and its relationship to other organs and biochemical processes mean that it quickly becomes vulnerable when the system is under strain. If the body is starved of the nutrients it needs, or conversely if it is overloaded with certain vitamins or minerals, then the skin starts to look pale and unhealthy and may eventually become prone to skin disorders.

The Anti-Acne Detox

Every day our bodies are bombarded with toxins, not only from the heavily processed foods in our diets, but also from the polluted atmosphere that surrounds us. Even fruits and vegetables often contain toxins, as modern farming methods involve the use of pesticides and other chemicals, so try to eat as much organic produce as possible or at least wash any fruit and vegetables before eating them. Processed foods are also chemically treated and this and other preserving processes alter the natural food, depleting it of many essential nutrients. Many food additives are toxic in high quantities.

We are also exposed to an increasing number of atmospheric pollutants from cars and industrial chemicals. Tobacco smoke pollutes the air and it contains a variety of poisonous heavy metals, such as cadmium. These clog up our skin pores and pass into our blood stream via our lungs. Even everyday cleaning products contain toxic substances and it is important to protect your skin by wearing rubber gloves in order to avoid over-exposure to these poisonous materials.

All these toxic substances have a cumulative effect on our health which is often reflected in the condition of our skin. The skin is an organ of detoxification and if its pores are blocked with dirt and grime it will not be able to carry out its job efficiently.

ACNE

Acne and other skin conditions often indicate that the body is in a state of toxic overload. This occurs when the body's organs of detoxification, namely the immune system, the liver, the lungs, the kidneys, the intestines, the bowel and the lymphatic system, are over-exposed to toxins and are unable to cope with them effectively. This causes a build-up of toxins in the body and the skin then comes to the rescue and attempts to eliminate them. Blemishes, pimples, boils or rashes on the skin are often a sign that the body is trying to rid itself of toxins.

If toxins in the body are not excreted efficiently, the system is put under pressure and symptoms like tiredness, lethargy, aches, pains and irritability as well as skin problems such as acne can be the result. A good way to cleanse the body of potentially harmful pollutants is to follow a specially designed detox programme. Once thought of just in terms of drug and alcohol rehabilitation, detoxing is an increasingly popular way of breaking bad eating habits and restoring energy levels. A detox diet consisting of raw fruits and whole grains has a number of other beneficial effects like helping the body to eliminate the cellulite that afflicts most women, and which is another indication of a build-up of toxins in the body.

In today's society, daily life is often busy and stressful and finding time for a detox regime can be a problem. To have a really effective detox, you will need to kick-start your body into eliminating the toxins present in your body by cutting out all toxins from your diet. You should drink large quantities of pure water and eat mainly raw fruit and vegetables and nothing else for a couple of days. This will encourage your body to detox, but all the benefits of this will be lost unless you continue to eat mainly raw foods for a further week or so and avoid all processed foods and stimulants such as tea, coffee and alcohol.

Embarking on such a detox programme is pretty daunting, and you will need to set aside a restful weekend in which to begin your detox. Stock your fridge and kitchen cupboards with

THE ANTI-ACNE DIET

a rich variety of fruit and vegetables and healthy brown rice, pulses and nuts before you start, so that all the good food you need is ready to hand. After a few days, white meat can be included; tofu is a good meat substitute for casseroles and sauces as it is a rich source of protein. It may be a good idea to remove all tempting toxic foods, such as chocolate and fatty dairy produce, from your kitchen altogether.

The healthier you are, the easier detoxing is, but no matter how fit you are, the detox can have some temporary side-effects, including nausea, headaches and lethargy, depending on the initial level of toxins in your body. Don't be put off; these symptoms don't last long. Remember not to attempt anything that requires exertion while detoxing. It wouldn't be sensible to begin it at the beginning of a hectic working week. Plan to start a detox at the weekend when you can just relax.

This detox programme begins with a twenty-four-hour period of fasting – the easiest time is from 7pm on Friday evening after a light meal, until 7pm the following day. If you feel fasting is out of the question you may want to start detoxing with raw fruits and vegetables for two days. On Saturday you can eat a single variety of fruit, for example apples, pears, grapes or melons. On Sunday include salad vegetables and on Monday you can add nuts, seeds, grains and vegetable broths. Remember to keep drinking pure water – aim for at least eight glasses a day.

THE DETOX

Day 1 – *drink pure water only (still mineral water or filtered water), and eat only a single variety of fruit.*

Day 2 – *carry on drinking plenty of water but now you can introduce raw fruits and salad vegetables.*

Day 3 – *as Day 2, plus nuts, seeds, well-cooked grains and vegetable broths. Steamed vegetables with brown rice is a simple and tasty meal which is also highly nutritious.*

Dairy products and wheat should be avoided for a further six weeks if you want to feel the full effects of the detox. Following a diet without bread, pasta, cereals, cheese, milk, etc may sound difficult, but plenty of alternatives can be found in health food shops and the rewards are high. Instead of eating toast for breakfast, try starting the day with organic muesli with fresh fruit. Baked potatoes with cottage cheese or tuna, or vegetable soups, make great lunches, and vegetable risottos and fish dishes are good, healthy evening meals. Soon, your energy levels will soar and while blemishes on the skin will not disappear straight away, over a period of time you will notice an improvement.

Skin-Saving Foods

A balanced diet made up of the right quantities of protein, fibre, vitamins and carbohydrates helps us to stay fit and active. Try and eat as much fresh and as little processed produce as possible. Far fewer people die of heart disease and cancer in developing countries, where the diet is usually based more on fresh meat, vegetables and fruit. A healthy diet is a life-saver as well as a skin-saver!

Plenty of fresh fruit and vegetables are essential for a clearer complexion, as are whole grains like brown rice and oats which provide fibre – the bulk that is required to keep things moving and flush out the system. Nuts and seeds like alfalfa, pumpkin and sunflower seeds are an important source of nutrients. Always use olive oil and sunflower oil for cooking. You don't have to become a vegetarian but it is important to cut down on fatty red meats and eat more chicken, game and fish (especially the oily varieties such as mackerel and herring). Drinking plenty of filtered or bottled mineral water and avoiding stimulants such as alcohol, tea and coffee also improves the condition of the skin.

THE ANTI-ACNE DIET

All nutrients work together to provide the energy and necessary raw materials for the constant rejuvenation and maintenance of each cell, organ and gland in the body so it is important to make sure that our diet provides a balance of all the food groups. The following is a simple guide, showing the foods that should be eaten daily, you can eat as much as you like of these. It's easy to follow and can be supplemented with meat and fish, dairy products and carbohydrates.

Whole grains	2 or more types
Fresh fruit	2 or more varieties
Vegetables	3 or more varieties (in addition to potatoes which are classified as a starchy food)
Unrefined oils	1 tablespoon
Herbs and spices	2 or more types

Internal Acne Tonic

Herbs are highly nutritious and there is a wealth of herbs which can help to cleanse our bodies and clear our skin. Here is a recipe for a really effective internal herbal tonic:

25g (1oz) blue flag – *boosts circulation and regulates bowel movements*
25g (1oz) echinacea – *immune-boosting and skin-healing*
25g (1oz) cleavers – *boosts the lymphatic system and is traditionally used for treating skin conditions*
25g (1 oz) figwort – *a kidney tonic and blood purifier which is used to treat chronic skin complaints.*

Blend the dried ingredients together and infuse in 600ml (1 pint) of almost boiling water. Drink three small cupfuls daily,

ACNE

after breakfast, lunch and dinner. The herbal extracts may be bought dried from a herbal supplier and made up daily.

Vitamin Finder

VITAMIN A

Often referred to as the 'skin vitamin', vitamin A is an important part of an anti-acne diet as it works to repair skin tissues. It also improves the vision and is vital to our immune system. There are two components of vitamin A: retinol, which is found in eggs, meat, fish, liver, and butter; beta-carotene, found in green and orange coloured vegetables like carrots, oranges, apricots, cabbage, spinach, etc. Beta-carotene acts as an antioxidant and controls free-radical activity. A deficiency of vitamin A can damage the process of normal cell repair and renewal and may eventually lead to a condition known as hyperkeratosis. This is when new cells die off before they reach the surface of the skin and collect with other debris and secretions, clogging up the oil sacs and follicles. The flow of the skin's natural oils and secretions is therefore restricted and acne, dandruff and more serious ailments such as conjunctivitis, styes and burning eyes can occur as a result.

THE VITAMIN B GROUP

There are more than a dozen vitamins in this group and all are closely interdependent. The richest sources of the B vitamins are unprocessed cereals, brown rice and whole grains, dairy produce, pulses, meat, fish and green vegetables. Vitamins B2 and B3 help to break down the fats, proteins and carbohydrates in the body and a lack of these vitamins can cause pellagra (rough skin). Vitamin B6 regulates the nervous system, metabolises the fats, proteins, minerals and essential fatty acids which help to fight inflammatory skin conditions. Other members of this family of vitamins include vitamins B9 and B12. One of vitamin B9's most important functions is to combat potential neurological birth defects in pregnant women, while B12 is concerned with preventing the development of nervous diseases.

Vitamin C

The most well known of all the vitamins, vitamin C is directly linked to the maintenance and repair of healthy skin cells and also helps to manufacture collagen, a principal body protein which supports the skin tissue. Deficiency in vitamin C can mean that wounds take longer to heal and the skin may become dry and chapped. Scurvy was once a common symptom of vitamin C deficiency. Vitamin C is also a powerful healer and acts as a cleanser, assisting the body in neutralising toxic substances and eliminating them from the body. Bioflavonoids are a group of vitamins found alongside vitamin C which maintain the intricate network of blood vessels and capillaries, and also work to combat inflammatory skin disorders. Vitamin C is found in most varieties of fresh fruit and vegetables. It can easily be destroyed by overcooking so it's always best to steam vegetables – if you want to boil them use just a small quantity of water. Pollution, stress, alcohol and smoking (even passive smoking) seriously deplete our levels of vitamin C – smoking only one cigarette wipes out the equivalent of the entire vitamin C content of an orange.

Vitamin D

Vitamin D is an unusual vitamin as it is synthesised naturally in the skin by exposing it to daylight, Vitamin D strengthens the skin tissue and keeps the complexion looking vibrant and fresh.

Vitamin E

Foods plentiful in this vitality or virility vitamin are whole grains (wheatgerm), eggs and unrefined vegetable oils. Food refining drastically lowers the vitamin E levels so cornflakes, for example, will lose 95 percent of this important nutrient. Working closely with vitamins A and C against the damaging activity of free radicals, vitamin E also has important antioxidant and cleansing properties which are helpful in maintaining a clear skin. As more research is conducted it is also becoming apparent that vitamin E seems to protect the essential fatty acids, vital ingredients in the structure of the skin. In addition vitamin E helps to ensure a healthy flow of blood to the surface of the skin by protecting the blood vessels, and acts as an anti-inflammatory agent by preventing the formation of leukotrines, hormone-like substances that occur naturally in the blood.

Minerals and Trace Elements

Minerals are another life-giving group of substances found in the body and they can be divided into two categories: those found in greater amounts, including calcium and sodium, and the trace elements which are present in smaller quantities, such as copper, sulphur and zinc. All are necessary to sustain normal healthy life and are essential in the battle against illness and infection.

Calcium and sodium are two of the better-known minerals. Calcium is found in milk and dairy products and is vital for the formation of healthy teeth and bones. The main drawback, though, is that a high intake of dairy products is mucus-forming, aggravating sinusitis, coughs, colds and respiratory problems. Found in most foods in the form of salt, sodium is the most ubiquitous mineral and, because nowadays we tend to eat more preserved and processed foods which all contain salt, deficiencies are rare. Together with potassium, salt helps to control the blood pressure, but too much of it ends up having the reverse effect, leading to the swelling of limbs and joints.

THE ANTI-ACNE DIET

Additionally, a diet with a high salt content may also intensify rosaceous acne. Magnesium and phosphorus are important trace elements which work with calcium to form teeth and bones. Plentiful in nuts, shrimps, soya beans, green leafy vegetables and whole grains, magnesium also assists in regulating the metabolism.

Of the trace elements, iron is the most well known, perhaps because deficiencies are commonplace, especially among women during menstruation. The Department of Health has reported that as many as 90 percent of teenage girls may be anaemic, or iron deficient. Although iron can be found in many fresh meats and vegetables, the chemical fertilisers used in modern farming methods deplete the iron content. It can also be difficult to absorb, especially if we eat lots of wheat-based products. Iron is the most essential component of haemoglobin, the red pigment in the blood both responsible for transmitting oxygen to the cells and forming part of the connective tissue that supports the skin. If we are anaemic our skin tends to look pale and sallow and may become vulnerable to rashes.

As we have seen, zinc and iodine have both been linked to acne: an excess of iodine can cause the skin to become inflamed, whereas depleted levels of zinc in the body tend to encourage the development of spots and acne. The other trace elements are copper, manganese, sulphur and selenium, all of which assist the metabolic process and contribute to the formation and renewal of cells. Selenium is a vigorous antioxidant, especially when combined with natural vitamin E. Fish, shellfish, heart, liver, kidney, avocados, garlic, onions, mushrooms, brewer's yeast and whole grains are all rich sources of selenium.

Taking vitamin and mineral supplements can improve acne-prone skin. Sufferers may benefit from taking extra amounts of zinc – about 30–40mg per day taken 1½ hours after eating and preferably at night. Acne linked to premenstrual tension (PMT) or the contraceptive pill may benefit from vitamin B-complex supplements, especially vitamin B6, while a small selenium supplement of 200mcg per day can help men suffering from acne. Those who are affected by acne rosacea can benefit from supplements of zinc, the B-complex vitamins and extra vitamin C. Small amounts of silicon and zinc can also help to protect the capillary walls and strengthen the immune system to resist infection.

Amino Acids

Amino acids are yet another group of nutrients vital for good health. Forming the basis of every kind of protein in our food, some twenty or so amino acids have been identified. Because the body is unable to manufacture twelve of these, these so-called essential amino acids have to be obtained through our diet. They are found in meat (game, pork and chicken), wheatgerm, oats, eggs and other dairy products. Scientific research is only beginning to touch on the functions of the amino acids, but two have been found to be particularly important to the skin. Present in beans, pulses, garlic, onions and eggs, methionine helps to regenerate collagen and is a significant anti-ager. Cysteine, on the other hand, acts as an antioxidant against the poisonous substances that we breathe in, such as metals and cigarette smoke, all of which are bad news for the skin as well as for our health in general.

Essential Fatty Acids

Dermatologists have recently paid a good deal of attention to a group of nutrients known as essential fatty acids. The EFAs can be divided into two groups: simply the good and the bad. The saturated fats are hard animal fats such as butter and lard and are major factors in contributing to heart disease. In the UK we still lag behind the Americans in reducing our intake of saturated fats. Polyunsaturated fats on the other hand, help to keep the skin supple and smooth. These come from vegetable and fish oils, and some fish oils have been prescribed to patients suffering from acne and psoriasis. The healing properties of fish oils were first discovered when it was found that Eskimos, whose diet is high in natural fish oil, didn't suffer from heart disease, diabetes or acne; however, some Eskimos living in Canada and eating a modern diet soon began to suffer from these disorders. Cod liver oil and fish oil supplements may help acne sufferers if taken regularly.

Enzymes

Destroyed by heat and food processing, enzymes can only be obtained by eating fresh, raw foods. For this reason it is essential that our diets incorporate plenty of salads and fresh fruit. The more unusual tropical fruits such as pineapple and papaya provide us with enzymes that are useful in repairing the damaged cells and tissues that can lead to inflammatory skin disorders. Other enzymes work to strengthen the collagen and elastin tissues which help to keep the skin firm and supple.

By being aware of what we eat and taking control of our diet we can reduce the severity of most forms of acne. We should ensure that all our hard work is not undone by drinking alcohol and smoking, and we should avoid caffeine, salt, saturated fats and sugar. Over the past decade there has been a significant increase in awareness of the links between diet and health and there is now a greater choice than ever before. Health food shops have sprung up in almost every town and village and most supermarkets are now responding to customer demands by stocking a variety of health foods, including organic and 'free

ACNE

range' produce. Since organic produce is derived from plants or animals raised without the use of hormones, pesticides or chemical fertilisers, 'going organic' gives us protection against the proven damaging effects of these substances. If you are really interested in eating well, get to know your local health food shop and pay close attention to the food you eat.

5

Clear Skin Care

How to care for the skin and what type of regime to follow is the subject of much discussion. Many women and a small, but rapidly increasing, number of men do follow a skincare routine – cleansing, toning and moisturising twice a day; first thing in the morning and last thing at night. Others, however, still choose to skip the daily grind and go for the soap and water option. Janet Bass, Group Leader in research and development at Elizabeth Arden says 'When you're dealing with a subject like skin, you're bound to get contradictions because it's highly individual.' The skin is an organ that is constantly changing, affected by factors such as age, hormones and the environment. Janet Bass's advice is to be flexible and to be prepared to change your skincare programme. Following a basic skincare routine and using products you are happy with has many benefits and helps to maintain a clear complexion.

For sufferers of acne, however, it is more important than ever to choose the right products and to have a consistent skincare routine. Mitchell S Wortzman, President of Neutrogena Dermatologics explains: 'Proper cleansing, toning and moisturising products are important to the acne patient, mainly because the improper choice of these products can cause irritation to the follicle and exacerbate existing acne conditions. The typical acne patient will often be using drying and/or irritating treatment products. Using cleansers which are too harsh or toners which are high in alcohol will continue to overdry the skin and create more inflammation. Proper moisturising is important because well-moisturised skin tends to be less prone

ACNE

to irritation. Products especially designed for sensitive skin, ie hypoallergenic products without perfumes or irritants or allergens, won't cure acne, but will make those treatments that do, better tolerated.'

Choosing Skincare Products

There is no magic potion that will make spots and blemishes disappear instantly. The results of a new skincare regime will take at least three weeks to show, as skin renewal takes between twenty-one and twenty-eight days. The answer is to follow an appropriate programme and use products that are suitable for skin affected by acne. It is always worth testing a new product on a hidden patch of skin first and waiting twenty-four hours to see how your skin reacts.

Acne sufferers should chose products that are hypoallergenic, which literally means less allergy provoking. Free from colourants and perfumes, these cosmetics are less likely to irritate problem skin. Studies show that 50 percent of all allergic reactions to skincare products are caused by fragrances. The remaining half are caused by preservatives, such as parabens and propylene glycol which irritate and inflame sensitive and problem skin. Unfortunately even hypoallergenic formulations often contain one or more of these substances, so it is best to check the ingredients carefully before you buy. Choose skincare products with added vitamins and therapeutic herbal extracts, such as echinacea and aloe vera. In all cases, it is worth buying skincare products which list their ingredients, so you know exactly what you are getting. This form of ingredient listing will become mandatory by law in 1998, but it is possible to find ethical companies who are already open about their ingredients.

Cleansing

The skin is a self-cleansing organ, so in an ideal world we wouldn't have to wash. Unfortunately dirt, pollution and make-up all mean that the skin becomes too blocked to cope by itself and following a skincare routine is essential to help it out. Without cleansing it would take twenty-five days on average for the skin to rid itself of the debris collected during the course of a normal modern day!

SOAP AND WATER

On the whole, washing the face with soap and water is not advisable for acne sufferers. Many soaps are made with animal fats such as tallow and tend to strip the skin of its natural oils, leaving it overly dry. Soaps also disturb the skin's delicate Ph balance, leaving it vulnerable to bacteria and infection until the balance is restored. Soap has an alkaline pH of around 8, whereas the skin is naturally slightly acidic with a pH of 5.5. Soap doesn't remove make-up effectively and often leaves a residue on the skin which causes further dryness unless it is rinsed off very thoroughly. It's not all bad news for those who cannot get themselves out of the soap and water habit though, as there are some soaps containing special ingredients to remove excess oils and bacteria which, unlike others, do not leave a drying residue behind. Look for those labelled as being suitable for sensitive skins.

CLEANSING CREAMS

Using a cleansing cream is a less risky and more effective way of clearing away the dirt and grime that collects on the skin on a daily basis. Cleansers are oil-in-water emulsions and clean the skin by dissolving the detritus and wiping it off the face. The first cleansing cream was invented by a Greek physician, Galen, who called his product cold cream because of its cooling sensation on the skin. If you wear make-up, removing it with cleansing cream or lotion is crucial. Most make-up is wax or oil based and therefore needs a wax/oil solution to remove it properly. Dr Chu of the Acne Support Group believes that cleansing the skin with the right product can be a great help in controlling the problem of acne.

For common acne problems he recommends Acnisal, a medicated cleanser that contains salicylic acid, which works by unclogging blocked sebaceous glands. Acnizal should not be used at the same time as any other hydroxy-acid products, such as alpha-hydroxy-acid (AHA) creams or face scrubs.

Wash-off creams and gels effectively combine both cream cleansing and the feel of a soap and water routine. Unlike soap and water, however, they treat the skin more gently and are non-irritating. Designed to wash off easily, these creams and gels are mainly water based and contain synthetic detergents which emulsify on contact with the epidermis. Choose the gentlest variants available, formulated for sensitive skins.

Toning

Step two of a daily skincare programme is to apply a toner or astringent. Contrary to popular belief, however, toners do not shrink the pores. If the pores have been enlarged by the overproduction of sebum, which can happen during teenage years, or if blackheads have developed, the pores can never return to their normal size. Toners create an illusion of shrinking the pore size by slightly inflaming the pores of an infected area which by comparison make the other pores appear smaller. Toners are an effective second cleanser, removing the final traces of dirt and oil from the face; they also soothe and soften the skin. Acne sufferers should be careful to choose a mild astringent and avoid those that contain alcohol. Some toners contain useful herbal extracts such as echinacea, comfrey and aloe vera. If you cannot find a toner that doesn't irritate your acne, it is possible to skip this second step and splash the skin with cool water instead.

Moisturising

Moisturising is the final step of the programme and it is essential for all skin types, especially in today's drying office atmospheres and with the use of central heating in most homes. Oily and acne-prone skins need as much protection against moisture loss and against the effects of bacteria as dry skins. Until recently, it was thought that acne could be alleviated by stripping the skin of its facial oils, but it has since been discovered that this only serves to stimulate the sebaceous glands into producing more sebum.

Moisturising creams and lotions work by forming a protective film over the epidermis. This both helps to seal the moisture in and also keeps potentially harmful bacteria out. The moisture content of each cell in the human body is 80 percent, while the amount of moisture in the air is only 1 percent in total. The skin is our only barrier against a constant loss of moisture. It produces its own natural moisturising factors (NMFs), a collection of compounds which boosts the levels of moisture in the cells. By applying moisturiser we can actively improve this biochemical process.

In addition, moisturising keeps the skin fresh and young looking by smoothing out lines and wrinkles. You may need to use different moisturising creams at different times; for example, during winter sebum production decreases and a richer cream might be required. Again, moisturisers formulated with added vitamins and natural herbal extracts are worth looking out for.

Skincare Programme for Acne

Some skincare programmes have been developed specifically for acne-prone skin, utilising a combination of skincare products and prescription treatments. The following is a good example.

Nightly
1. Remove eye make-up with a non-oily cleanser.
2. Work up a lather with a bar of soap and warm water and spread over your face. Wash thoroughly but gently.
3. Rinse off all the soap with ten handfuls of warm water.
4. Allow your face to dry naturally.
5. Spread a layer of prescription antibiotic lotion all over your face, not just on areas of acne.

Daily
1. With warm water, work up a lather with a bar of soap and spread over your face. Wash gently.
2. Rinse off the soap with five handfuls of warm water.
3. Allow your face to dry thoroughly.
4. Apply a thin layer of prescription antibiotic lotion.
5. Apply an oil-free, non-medicated foundation if desired.

You can also cleanse your skin during the day with a mild astringent and then reapply the antibiotic lotion.

SKINCARE ADDITIONS
The basic cleansing, toning and moisturising routine can be supplemented with other skincare treatments which keep the skin looking clear and fresh. Exfoliation, using a facial scrub or grains (usually pumice or nut kernels), helps the skin to get rid of dead cells which can block the pores and hair follicles. Each day the body sheds some 500 million skin cells and by using a

gentle scrub we can increase the blood circulation in the dermis which effectively stimulates the development of new cells. Experts now believe that regular exfoliation every other day should be integrated into a basic skincare regime. However, sufferers of acne should be careful not to rub too harshly and should choose a gentle scrub; one based on oatmeal is a good idea. You can make your own scrub by blending the juice of a grapefruit with three to four tablespoons of oatmeal. Grind into a fine paste and leave it on the skin for fifteen minutes before removing with warm water. Work the scrub over the face while you are washing.

Spot zappers
For sufferers of mild acne there are a number of effective spot-zapping products available. Some of the most effective on-the-spot treatments contain essential oils to be used neat on spots and pimples (see Chapter 3). Milk of magnesia is effective at drying up pustules, while neat vodka is also an effective spot zapper. Simply dab on to the affected areas using a cotton bud.

Face and body masks
Face and body masks, applied once or twice weekly, are another good addition to any skincare programme. Both relaxing and reviving, face masks have been used as a beauty treatment for centuries. Noblewomen in Rome made masks from ground asparagus roots and goat's milk, which were rubbed into the skin with pieces of warm bread. Unfortunately, this treatment did nothing to counter the effects of wearing the fashionable but highly toxic lead paste on the faces. Some face masks moisturise the face; others, such as masks based on kaolin or Fuller's earth, are more suitable for oily skin. They work by drawing the oil and dirt away from the skin via the surface tension created by the mask and the facial skin, leaving it bright and fresh.

ACNE

Anti-acne face pack

This recipe for a face pack can be used on the body as well, as the back is another prime area for acne:

- 100g (4oz) Fuller's earth
- 2 egg whites, lightly beaten
- 1 teaspoon (5ml) alum crystals
- 1 teaspoon (5ml) sulphur powder
- 6 drops of tea tree essential oil

Mix together the Fuller's earth and lightly beaten egg whites until they form a smooth paste (add a few drops of cold water if the mixture becomes too hot to handle). Add the alum crystals (available from the chemist), sulphur powder and tea tree essential oil and stir well to combine all the ingredients. Apply to the face and ask a friend or partner to massage the mixture into the back. Any leftover mixture may be used on the feet to smooth and soften hard skin. Leave the pack to dry completely (approximately fifteen minutes) before rinsing away with tepid water in the shower and gently patting the skin dry.

Facial saunas

Facial saunas can be used prior to applying a face mask. Steaming helps to loosen the dirt and grease in the pores, as well as opening them up and allowing the mask to penetrate more effectively. Alternatively, you can make your own herbal steam bath with hot infusions of lavender, yarrow or chamomile – flowers which, herbalist Nalda Gosling suggests, are particularly successful in combating acne. Simply pour ¾ pint (500ml) of hot water into a bowl over a handful of flowers, cover your head with a towel and lean over the bowl. Steam the face for five to ten minutes each day.

SKIN CARE FOR MEN

The cleansing, toning and moisturising ritual is predominantly associated with women's skin care. However, men too can benefit from following a skincare programme, especially if they have skin disorders. Men's skin is thicker, oilier, has more collagen and elastin and has larger pore openings that become blocked with dirt and oil. Men also have to contend with shaving. In *Fast Forward*, the journal published by the Acne Support Group, two male acne sufferers described two different ways of dealing with the painful process of shaving. The first found he could benefit from a wet shave with a sensitive-skin shaving foam using quick downward strokes. The second used a sensitive-skin shaving gel and showered after the shave to soothe his skin. After drying he used an after-shave gel and rich moisturising cream to stop his skin from becoming overly dry. If acne makes shaving uncomfortable it may be helpful to experiment with different methods. Shaving can be a problem if you suffer from acne, as the skin is often already sore and inflamed and shaving exacerbates this. A razor can slice off the top of spots and shaving creams can irritate sensitive skin.

American dermatologist, Nelson Lee Novick, recommends using an electric razor on the lightest setting, as this has a less irritating effect and the chances of nicking and cutting the skin are lower. Shave more rather than less, and use a cream specially designed for sensitive skin.

Some men may be tempted to grow a beard to hide their acne, but the thick covering of hair will make the underlying skin warm and moist – the perfect breeding ground for bacteria. Beards also prevent air reaching and healing the acne. If you do suffer from acne, make sure that you wash any facial hair frequently.

Washing the face with a cleansing product can help to remove the dirt, dead cells and excess oil or sebum, all of which encourage fresh outbreaks of spots. Men suffering from acne should choose products that are non-irritating. Men should also use moisturisers, such as a lightweight lotion that nourishes the skin with added vitamins and herbal extracts.

Hair Care

Hair products can also cause problems with facial skin, especially around the hairline. As much care should be taken over the products we use for our hair as those we use on our skin, as certain hair products containing lanolin can aggravate oil problems and cause 'pomade acne' on the forehead and the temples. Use a mild shampoo and conditioner and ensure that you rinse them out thoroughly. Take care with styling products such as mousses and setting gels as many of these contain alcohol which can dry and irritate the skin.

Try making your own shampoo which is gentle on the skin and is suitable for all hair types. Here is a recipe.

Sandalwood and soapwort shampoo

25g (1oz) chopped soapwort root
25g (1oz) dried chamomile flowers
250ml (8fl oz) hot water
20 drops sandalwood essential oil

Place the chopped soapwort root and the dried chamomile flowers in a bowl and pour on the almost boiling water. Stir, cover and leave overnight. In the morning strain well and add the essential oil. Use just a small amount of the shampoo each time.

DIY Skin Care

Making and using your own cosmetics is a fun, cheap and, more importantly, a natural way to treat your skin. Using ingredients such as herbs, fruit and vegetables, you can prepare many different infusions, astringents and creams that can both treat skin problems and minimise the risk of irritation caused by the harmful chemicals and preservatives found in many manufactured products.

CLEAR SKIN CARE

You will find you probably already have many ingredients in the kitchen, such as honey, cornflour, olive oil, corn oil and oatmeal, for example. Other raw materials such as aloe vera juice, hazelnut oil and evening primrose oil are widely available from supermarkets, chemists or health food stores. No special equipment is needed, although it is best to keep a set of utensils for the purpose, separate from the ones you use for cooking, to reduce the risk of cross-contamination of germs and odours. With homemade recipes using fresh fruit and vegetables it is important to remember that they will have a lifespan of only a few days and must be stored in the fridge to keep them fresh.

Be careful to keep the products out of direct sunlight and, for water-based formulations, only use filtered, boiled and cooled water or distilled water available from the chemist. Remember to wash your hands before starting.

RECIPES

A homemade gently medicated soap bar is excellent for using on oily, acne-prone complexions. The essential oils purify the skin and have a gentler effect than many commercial soaps.

Gently medicated soap

150g (5oz) soft olive oil soap
50ml (2fl oz) strong sage tea
10 drops tea tree essential oil
10 drops lavender essential oil
1tsp almond or jojoba oil (to grease the moulds)

Make the sage tea by infusing a dessertspoonful of dried sage in a cup of almost boiling water. Chop or grate the olive oil soap into small pieces. Place this soap in a small saucepan and begin to melt over a high heat. Add the sage tea and stir thoroughly. Remove from the heat and allow to cool before adding the essential oils, as heat reduces their strength. Pour the mixture into greased bun tins or egg cups and leave in a cool place to

ACNE

harden overnight. Remove from the moulds using a sharp knife and wrap in tissue paper.

Tea tree oil spot buster
5ml (1tsp) hazelnut or jojoba oil
2 drops tea tree essential oil
Piece of muslin cloth or face flannel

First soften your spots by dipping the cloth into hot water and allowing it to cool on your face, then repeat the process. Mix the oils in the palm of one hand and apply to the affected area with warm fingertips. Massage gently to bring fresh blood supplies to the surface of the skin, which will help carry trapped toxins away from beneath the skin. Leave overnight.

Oily, acne-prone skin can be enhanced by using a light, oil-free moisturiser. Make your own by following the recipe below.

Oil-free moisturiser
20g linseeds
200 ml (7fl oz) boiling water
15ml (1tbsp) glycerine
15ml (1tbsp) rosewater
1 drop neroli essential oil (optional)

Linseeds are a good source of mucilage, a gel-like paste that soothes the skin. Crack the linseeds open by whizzing in a blender or coffee grinder for a few seconds. Transfer them to a small cup and pour on the boiling water. Stir continually while the linseeds steep as the mixture cools down. Strain off the linseeds and discard, retaining the liquid.

Mix in the linseed with the glycerine and rosewater to form a light moisturising lotion. Add the neroli essential oil to give the lotion a wonderful aroma of orange blossom.

CLEAR SKIN CARE

Men who suffer from acne will probably find that many commercial shaving products can irritate and inflame the condition. Home-made cucumber shaving cream is an excellent solution. Containing cucumber juice to soothe the skin, lavender oil to heal any razor nicks, and natural plant oils, it leaves the skin moisturised and smooth. Try the following recipe.

Cucumber shaving cream
175g (6oz) coconut oil
50ml (2fl oz) witchhazel
90ml (6tbsp) almond oil
15ml (1tbsp) cucumber juice
4 drops sandalwood essential oil
4 drops lavender essential oil

Melt the coconut oil slowly in a small saucepan over a low heat. Remove from the heat and stir in the witchhazel and almond oil. Make the cucumber juice by blending half a peeled cucumber and passing the liquid through a fine sieve. Add the juice to the mixture together with the sandalwood and lavender essential oils. Mix thoroughly and pour into a jar.

To use, stir the cream with the fingertips and apply to the skin. After shaving, remove any remaining traces of cream with a hot damp flannel and pat the skin dry.

Cosmetic Care

Following a skincare programme which nourishes problem skin and treats the acne-infected areas helps to revitalise the skin's condition. In addition, with the right cosmetics and techniques to camouflage spots and redness, acne sufferers can feel less self-conscious about facing the world. Accentuating features like the eyes and lips detracts attention from spots and blemishes. When choosing cosmetics stay away from oily foundations and

ACNE

perfumed products. In general look for ranges that are hypoallergenic and formulated with ingredients that are designed not to aggravate the skin.

Additionally, there are a number of cosmetic techniques that can be used to conceal facial areas affected by the blemishes and redness of acne. For those who suffer only mild symptoms, matt foundations of beige, tawny or olive colours underneath the final choice of shade can help to tone down the redness. Areas that are more red and infected can be improved by using foundations with green colours and corrective green base creams. The green pigment absorbs any red light, countering the reflection from red skin. Sufferers who have widespread acne rosacea need to use a pale green corrective camouflage product before applying the general foundation. Take care to blend and shade carefully, but if you're not sure about the products and techniques you are using you can always seek advice from a professional cosmetic camouflager. Dermablend produce an excellent range of waterproof camouflage creams (used by make-up artists to hide scars and birthmarks). For more information and details on where to buy, see Useful Addresses.

Glossary

Allantoin – a chemical extracted from the comfrey plant that stimulates cell division and therefore speeds up scar formation and aids the healing process of skin tissue.

Antibiotic – a substance that inhibits the growth of, or destroys, micro-organisms which can cause infection.

Anti-inflammatory – a substance that reduces inflammation of the tissues, so reducing pain and swelling. Some anti-inflammatory agents also work by stimulating the circulation.

Antioxidant – a substance which prevents the formation of destructive free radicals within the body and skin.

Antiseptic – a substance which fights infections and germs on the surface of the skin. All essential oils found in herbs are antiseptic to a varying degree.

Aromatherapy – the therapeutic use of essential oils to treat many kinds of disorders, notably skin complaints.

Astringent – any substance which causes a contraction of body tissue when applied to the skin.

Bacteria – a group of single-celled micro-organisms, commonly known as germs, some of which cause disease.

Collagen – main component of the connective tissue in the skin's dermis.

ACNE

Cyst – an abnormal lump or swelling, filled with fluid or semi-solid material, that may occur in any organ or tissue.

Dermabrasion – removal of the surface layer of the skin by high-speed sanding to improve the appearance of scars.

Dermatitis – inflammation of the deeper layers of skin.

Dermatologist – a medical specialist concerned with the diagnosis and treatment of skin disorders.

Detoxifying – eliminating toxins from the body.

Herbalism – the use of plants and herbs to treat a wide range of disorders.

Homoeopathy – a safe and effective treatment based on the principle that a substance causing the symptoms of an illness can be used in minute doses to relieve the same symptoms.

Hormones – substances created within the body by the various glands in the endocrine system. Used to regulate numerous bodily functions.

Keloid – an overgrowth of fibrous scar tissue following a trauma to the skin.

Lymphatic system – a system of vessels that drains lymph from all over the body into the blood stream. This system is part of the immune system, playing a major part in the body's defences against infection.

Pitting – formation of depressed scars following acne.

GLOSSARY

Sebaceous glands – glands in the skin that produce an oily substance called sebum. Some parts of the skin have many sebaceous glands while others have very few.

Sebum – the fatty secretion produced by the sebaceous glands which lubricates the hair and skin.

Stimulant – any substance which increases the power of the body to boost strength and energy.

Testosterone – the most important of the androgen hormones (male sex hormones). Testosterone stimulates bone and muscle growth and sexual development. It is produced by the testes in men and in very small amounts by female ovaries.

Tonic – invigorates and tones the body and promotes well-being.

Vitamins – over a dozen essential nutrients that the body cannot make from other substances and which must be supplied through diet.

Useful Addresses

The Acne Support Group
PO Box 230
Hayes UB4 9HW

British Complementary Medicine Association
St Charles Hospital
Exmoor Street
London W10 6DZ
Tel: 0181 964 1206

British Homoeopathic Association
27a Devonshire Street
London W1N 1RJ
Tel: 0171 935 2163

Dermablend
Gemini House
Flex Meadow
Harlow
Essex CM19 5TJ
Tel: 01279 421555

General Council and Register of Consultant Herbalists
Grosvenor House
40 Sea Way
Middleton-on-Sea
West Sussex PO22 7SA
Tel: 01326 317321

Homoeopathic Remedies
Nelson's Pharmacies Ltd
73 Duke Street
London W1M 6BY

International Federation of Aromatherapists
Department of Continuing Education
Royal Masonic Hospital
London W6 0TN

Potters Herbal Suppliers Ltd
Douglas Works
Leyland Mill Lane
Wigan
Lancashire WN1 2JB

Index

A
A, vitamin 56, 62
Addresses 87-8
Adult acne 18-21
Aggravating factors 17
Aloe vera 44, 70, 73
Amino acids 66
Antibiotics 39, 83
　　oral 27-8, 31
　　topical 27
Aromatherapy 47-50, 83
　　see also herbs

B
B, vitamin 62-3, 66
Bowel 40-1, 58
Burns 12
Burdock 44-5

C
C, vitamin 56, 63, 66
Cabbage 45
Calendula 45
Career woman acne 19-20
Causes 16
Chamomile 45, 48
Chemical peeling 33-4
Cleansing 71-2
Clindamycin 28
Collagen injections 34
Concealers 81-2

Contraceptive pill 15, 27-8, 29, 30, 65
Cosmetics, homemade 75, 78-81
Creams 25-7, 28-9, 31-2, 71-2
Cryotherapy 35

D
D, vitamin 54, 63
Dandelion 45
Dermabrasion 33, 84
Dermis 13-14
Detox
　　diet 57-60
　　process 39, 40-4
Dianette 29
Diet 17, 39-40, 53-68
Dry skin acne 19

E
E, vitamin 63-4
Echinacea 45-6, 70, 73
Enzymes 67-8
Epidermis 12
Erythromycin 28
Eskimos 67
Essential fatty acids 66-7
Exercise 44, 54
Exfoliation 14, 72, 74-5

89

F

Face
　mask 75
　pack 76
　sauna 47, 76
Fennel 46
Food
　see diet, nutrients, trigger foods

G

Garlic 43, 46-7
Gels 31-2
Glossary 83-5
GP, attitude of 36-7
Grades 17-18

H

Hair care 77-8
Herbs 44-7, 61-2
　see also aromatherapy
Homeostasis 40-4
Homeopathy 50-1, 84
Hormone replacement therapy 15

I

Ice pick scars 32-3
Injections
　collagen 34
　steroid 35
Intestines 41, 58
Isotretinoin 29-30

J

Juniper 48

K

Keloid scars 34-6, 84
Kidneys 41-2, 44, 58

L

Lavender 47, 48-9
Liver 42, 44, 58
Lotions 31-2
Lungs 42-3, 58
Lymphatics 43, 55, 58, 84

M

Masks 75
Medication
　over-the-counter 25-6
　prescription 27-8
Men 66, 76-7, 80-1
Minerals 64-6
Moisturising 73, 80
Myrrh 49
Myths 21-3

N

Nutrients, essential 56-7, 62-6

P

Patchouli 49
Peeling, chemical 33-4
Pitted scars 32-3, 84

R

Recipes 44-50, 61, 76, 78, 79-81
Retin-A 28-9
Rhinophyma 20
Rosacea acne 20-1, 51, 66
Rosemary 47

S

Sandalwood 49
Sauna, facial 47, 76
Scars 18, 32-6, 44
Scrubs
　see exfoliation
Sharks 52
Shaving 77, 80-1
Skin
　and exercise 44, 54
　as detoxifier 39, 43-4, 57-8
　brushing 43-4
　care 69-82
　food 60-1
　function 10-11
　life cycle 14-15
　structure 12-14
Soap 71, 79
Steaming
　see sauna
Steroids 35
Stress 19-20, 54
Sun 12, 15, 29, 54
Surgery, cosmetic 33-6

T

Tablets 27-8, 31
Tea tree oil 49-50, 80
Tetracycline 27
Thrush 27-8, 39
Tonic, internal 61-2
Toning 72-3
Trace elements 64-6
Treatment
　conventional 25-37
　natural 39-52
　new, 30, 52
Trigger foods 20, 54-6
Trimethoprim 28
Type 18-21

V

Vitamins 62-4, 85
Vulgaris, acne 9, 50-1

HOW TO ORDER YOUR BOXTREE BOOKS BY LIZ EARLE

Liz Earl's Quick Guides

Available Now
- [ ] 1 85283 542 7   Aromatherapy   £3.99
- [ ] 1 85283 544 3   Baby and Toddler Foods   £3.99
- [ ] 1 85283 543 5   Food Facts   £3.99
- [ ] 1 85283 546 X   Vegetarian Cookery   £3.99
- [ ] 0 7522 1619 8   Evening Primrose Oil   £3.99
- [ ] 0 7533 1614 7   Herbs for Health   £3.99
- [ ] 1 85283 984 8   Successful Slimming   £3.99
- [ ] 1 85283 989 9   Vitamins and Minerals   £3.99
- [ ] 1 85283 979 1   Detox   £3.99
- [ ] 0 7522 1635 X   Hair Loss   £3.99
- [ ] 0 7522 1636 8   Youthful Skin   £3.99
- [ ] 0 7522 1680 5   Healthy Pregnancy   £3.99
- [ ] 0 7522 1636 8   Dry Skin and Eczema   £3.99
- [ ] 0 7522 1641 4   Cod Liver Oil   £3.99
- [ ] 0 7522 1626 0   Juicing   £3.99

Coming Soon
- [ ] 0 7522 1645 7   Beating Cellulite   £3.99
- [ ] 0 7522 1673 2   Food Combining   £3.99
- [ ] 0 7522 1690 2   Post-natal Health   £3.99
- [ ] 0 7522 1675 9   Food Allergies   £3.99
- [ ] 0 7522 1685 6   Healthy Menopause   £3.99
- [ ] 0 7522 1668 6   Beating PMS   £3.99
- [ ] 0 7522 1663 5   Antioxidants   £3.99

ACE Plan Titles
- [ ] 1 85283 518 4   Liz Earle's Ace Plan
  The New Guide to Super Vitamins
  A, C and E   £4.99
- [ ] 1 85283 554 0   Liz Earle's Ace Plan
  Weight-Loss for Life   £4.99

All the books shown opposite are available at your local bookshop or can be ordered direct from the publisher. Just tick the titles you want and fill in the form below. Prices and availability subject to change without notice.

Boxtree Cash Sales,
PO Box 11, Falmouth, Cornwall TR10 9EN

Please send cheque or postal order for the value of the book(s), and add the following for postage and packing:

UK including BFPO – £1.00 for one book, plus 50p for the second book, and 30p for each additional book ordered up to a £3.00 maximum.
Overseas including Eire – £2.00 for the first book, plus £1.00 for the second book, and 50p for each additional book ordered.

OR
please debit this amount from my Access/VISA card (delete as appropriate)

Card number ☐☐☐☐☐☐☐☐☐☐☐☐☐☐☐☐☐☐☐☐

Amount £ ....

Expiry date on card ....

Signed ....

Name ....

Address ....

....

....